COVID Long- Hauler:

My Life Since COVID

Salam Kabbani

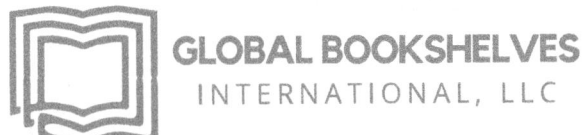

GLOBAL BOOKSHELVES
INTERNATIONAL, LLC

Table of contents

Dedication

For my mom. You brighten my world with sunshine when it's nothing but storms outside. I love you more than these three words could ever describe.

In loving memory of my cousin Eyad. You were one of COVID's first victims, a very young and healthy 32. You are gone, but you will never be forgotten.

Prologue

This is a memoir of my life since I was diagnosed with COVID.[1] I say since, not after, because this book is being written at a time when I am still dealing with post-acute sequelae of SARS-CoV-2 (PASC)[2-10]— also known as long-COVID, post-COVID conditions, or long-hauler syndrome. I will use these terms interchangeably throughout the book for ease of understanding.

I am a clinical pharmacist. I will not be providing any medical advice or information in this book. Some of my symptoms resolved with medications; however, I will not share the medications because I do not know who will be reading my book. A medication that helped me may be contraindicated for someone else and harm them instead. If you are experiencing any COVID or long-COVID symptoms,[11] please contact your primary care provider for medical advice. If you or a loved one are experiencing suicidal thoughts or ideation due to

COVID, please call the suicide prevention lifeline, which is available 24/7, at 800-273-8255. Starting July 16, 2022, everyone in the United States can call, text, or chat at 988 to be connected to the lifeline.

Additionally, I will talk about approximately how many COVID survivors are likely to experience PASC symptoms. The literature currently shows a wide range of 5%-80% of COVID survivors. These are all estimates based on current literature, which is very scant. You may be reading this book 10 years from now and the data may look very different, so please do not use this book as a medical reference, because it is not.

My story is unique to me. Some of you may have been experiencing PASC for longer than I have, and it may be worse for you. To that, I say that I am deeply sorry, and I hope you eventually improve. Some of you may have never gotten COVID, and to that I say kudos. Others may relate with some parts, and not so much with others. No matter, I hope you find some joy and benefit in this recounting of my long-COVID life.

I am sharing my story because I want all the long-haulers out there to know that you are not alone. You are seen and you are heard and you matter. And together we will get through this, no matter how long it takes. One of my all-time favorite fable twists coined anonymously is the saying, "This too shall pass. It may pass like a kidney stone, but it will pass." This is how I feel daily, living with PASC.

Introduction

"If you want to make God laugh, tell Him about your plans." –Woody Allen

This is the new tagline of my life journey. I am obsessed with the field of infectious diseases, and because of that, I am EXTRA cautious about getting any type of infection and spreading germs. So, you can imagine my excitement when I first heard about boosters becoming approved eight months after the second dose. I mean, I had gotten my second dose January 8, 2021, and this was sometime in late August, so I was ecstatic that I would be one of the first people to get an extra boost to my immunity. After all, I am a front-line warrior, so getting that booster is both necessary and altruistic, because it allows me to serve others while protecting myself and them from the virus.

I was working on a Saturday and helping someone in the drive-thru who revealed he had left the hospital against medical advice (AMA) and was COVID-positive. This patient informed me of this after he had given me all his paper scripts, and his mask had been down the whole time. Of course, I started panicking. I cannot tell you the amount of stress I started to feel knowing I was now in danger; not to mention so were my employees. So, after the patient left, I did everything shy of burning the place down to ensure we were properly sanitized again, and of course, his scripts were quarantined once they were scanned into the system.

About an hour after I had seen that patient, I started feeling some chills, but I figured it could have just been the stress of my interaction with a COVID-positive patient.

On Monday, I was having an incessant cough, and I remember explicitly telling my patients and employees, "Don't worry, it's not COVID, it's just the smoke from all the fires around us". For reference, I live in northern California, so every summer we are surrounded by wildfires that render our cars and lungs ash-filled reservoirs.

That afternoon, I heard my then-store manager talking about how one of our own employees tested positive, and how he was not going to tell anyone due to patient privacy. Now this, of course, was a load of crap, because any person who has been exposed to COVID has the right to know they've been exposed. It is especially important for contact tracing. So, I did my due diligence as a pharmacy manager, went back to the pharmacy, and told everyone to get tested, especially because said employee's vaccination status was unknown, and our front-end management did not enforce masks covering the nose.

The next day I was at home, unsuspectingly enjoying my day off, when I started to get some nasty chills. I figured, hey why not just be sure and do an antigen test — after all, I often find myself eating lunch in the breakroom with several employees, so better to be safe than sorry. Well, my test was positive, and thus began the longest journey of my life.

In this book, I plan to share my COVID story. Some of it will be pure facts. A lot of it will be my emotions and feelings up until now, because yes, dear reader, as I write this, I am still suffering from long-COVID and on disability. You will hear my perspective both as a healthcare worker and as a patient. I am writing this book because I know that I am one of MANY individuals impacted by the SARS-CoV-2 virus, and I want you to know that you are not alone. It may seem like it. I know I often feel that way, because long-COVID is a capricious beast that sneaks up on you when you least expect it. But you aren't alone. I hope this book feels like a warm hug and makes you feel seen and heard.

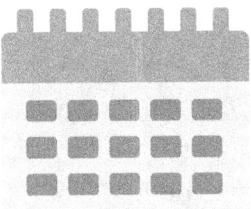

Chapter 1 : September 2021

The Quarantine

I tested positive on August 31, 2021. I thought this was going to be a 10-dayer —just like everyone else at the time — and then I would be back on my feet. Although I live in the same city as my parents, my mom was on the other coast with my grandma who was hospitalized with pneumonia at the time and my dad was also out of town — so all around, the timing was 10/10.

I don't recall the first few days being that horrible. In fact, I remember being able to go about my at-home activities fairly normally. Then things changed, and I started to deteriorate very quickly. I had several days where I could not talk because my voice was mostly gone, and it hurt that much to say anything. The chills that presented before I tested positive kept worsening and, to be honest, are still with me as I write these words in February 2022. Everything was hurting. To make matters worse, two of my employees also tested positive, so I was worried about what was going to be facing me back at work upon my return. My pharmacy has just shy of 500 scripts to fill every day — which is a high volume for reference — on top of anywhere from 70-150 vaccines per day and sometimes upwards of 50 COVID tests per day. So, you can imagine the added stress of knowing what was awaiting me. In addition, this was right around the time the first booster shots were going to be approved for the public. So, I knew I had to regain my health in 10 days because when I went back, I was going to roll up my sleeves and hit the ground running.

Except things kept getting worse. No amount of cough syrup was making my cough better. I was definitely taking more of my prescription cough medication than I was supposed to, but nothing seemed to touch my cough. My oxygen saturation never really dropped below 94% and even when it did, thankfully, it wasn't ongoing. But, my chest and lungs ached when I was breathing, when I was lying down, when I walked — pretty much when I did anything. I never spiked a true fever, but the ongoing chills were exhausting.

The best part was two weeks of uninterrupted diarrhea. I mean guys, when it rains, it pours. And if you are wondering, the pun is always intended. Of course, this was accompanied by some nausea and vomiting, as well as severe fatigue and muscle pain. Naturally, as my symptoms progressed, my provider extended my quarantine to 14 days, which gave me some hope for recovery before returning to work. At the time, the CDC guidance was to quarantine for 10 days, but my provider wanted to be sure I wasn't contagious since my symptoms were really bad.

Things No One Tells You

Being quarantined for 14 days sounds pretty straightforward, right? WRONG.

* If you don't have a washing machine at home, you run out of clean underwear very quickly. So, you end up having to spend money on express shipping for new undies, and then you feel gross wearing them without washing them first, but really, what's the alternative?

* You also have to buy clean towels. Unless you are super rich and bougie — and if you are, please adopt me and pay off my student loans — you probably don't have enough towels to circle 40 days. Okay, I didn't shower every day for 40 days because I was pretty much disabled, but let's say on average five days a week... That's a whopping 28.57 towels. I have about six and I'd like to think that's average. So yeah, my dad dropped off a few clean ones once he was back in town, but then I had to order more. Now, I wasn't quarantined for 40 days, but I had no strength to carry a laundry hamper — or anything else really — to go to my parent's house and do laundry. My mom was across the country during all of this. As selfish and needy as I wanted to be, I recognized that my hospitalized grandma that speaks no English was in more need of my mom's company than me, so she was

with her. And if you are wondering why my cardiologist dad who seems to work 24/7 didn't do my laundry ... Whooo buddy, we need to have a serious discussion about realistic expectations on the work-life balance of physicians. Anyhow the towels were bought, the lady was able to stay clean, and the laundry hamper casually expanded into empty grocery bags that were being temporarily stored in the linen closet.

* You spend a ton of money on services such as DoorDash, because how else are you going to get food delivered to your door? In my case, both my parents were out of town initially, and while I have the kindest neighbor on the planet, I was not going to give her a grocery list. Especially because when your body has its own gastrointestinal-palooza going on, one day you may be eating normally and the next you may not be able to stomach anything but yogurt and pudding. A fickle body like that is surely not going to trouble anyone with a constantly-evolving grocery list.

* Now, here is the kicker. When you live in an apartment complex, where do you throw out your trash? If you open your door, you very well may run into a neighbor and expose them. When you go to throw away the trash, even if you are wearing gloves, you are touching the same lid that everyone else is, so you still have a chance of exposing them. You can't put your trash in your backyard area because you live in Humboldt County and bears will literally come into your backyard and tear into that bag. So, what do you

do? You store all your trash inside one of your bathrooms for 14 days and keep the fan on to air out the smell. I mean ... how luxurious is this sounding? Okay, shark tank idea: I'm thinking we open a spa with these features and call it ... wait for it ... "The COVID Experience." I really wish I had taken a picture for the brochure right around now, but we can just be creative with our words guys, we are a team. But on a real note, for people who only have one bathroom in their household, this can become a serious problem. I don't know what the best solution is, but if you were or are in that position, I am sorry, and I applaud you for making it out of the trenches alive.

* You need a pet to survive. Okay, maybe that's my exaggerated opinion; however, as much cattitude as my Luna has, having something furry and purry cuddled up next to me in my darkest hours was one of the most comforting feelings I could possibly have. I also realize I'm very lucky that I chose to have a cat and not a dog, because seriously, if you live in an apartment building by yourself, how do you take your dog out every day and not break the quarantine? Luckily, I did not have to deal with that problem, but my heart goes out to all the dogs and their owners who did. I know, it's always the dogs that suffer.

* You have to accept eating what you can. By this, I mean that even if you are able to tolerate complete meals, you may not have the energy to cook yourself anything. If you don't have friends or family nearby to

cook for you, the reality is that you just need to get by. So, you might eat a banana and string cheese or microwaved macaroni and cheese for five days straight, and that's okay. Well, why don't you order Chipotle? I mean, I love a burrito bowl just as much as the next person, but I didn't want to eat anything store-bought at that point; at least not until my head was above the water again. I know I was already infected, but it's just how I was feeling at the time. And for those of you who have someone close to you who is going through this, please be a standup person and cook for them if you can. They are going to be too embarrassed to ask you, but really think about it ... do they need your help? Yeah, I'm betting $10 — because that's all I can afford — that they do. Now I will say I never lost my sense of taste or smell through this entire crapstorm, something I thank God for every day, because if you know me, you know I love food. Ironically, in early March, I had a day when my sense of taste really dulled out, but it was very short-lived. For those of you who experienced that symptom, I'm sorry; however, I cannot speak to that experience. I do know there are videos out there on TikTok where people describe what it's like if you are looking to learn more, or to simply not feel alone.

Cost of Living Through COVID

Okay, so we've been keeping score, right? Undies, food delivery services, medications, towels, audiobooks (more on that later). So those are all things I don't normally budget for because I can drive myself to the grocery store, pick up my own medications, and wash and reuse undergarments and towels. The audiobooks, on the other hand, I can't defend, because yes, I read that much. So how, you ask, did I afford to survive through this while being unemployed?

The first 80 hours were paid by my employer, as I was very fortunate to get COVID before September ended. Let me explain the reasoning to those of you living outside our majestic state of California — The law that mandates 80-hours of COVID pay ended on September 30th, 2021. As you can imagine, boy did I feel like I hit the jackpot with my timing. I mean, come on, if you are going to get COVID, you might as well hope to get the timing right, and that is exactly what happened.

Okay, but Salam, you're supposed to be good at math, you're a pharmacist … 80 hours is like two weeks … What about the other four weeks? This is where state disability kicks in.

Now I will humbly express my incompetence in any disability knowledge outside the state of California, so please do not use this book as your source of information for disability benefits. What I can tell you is the process is crummy, and that's sugar-coating it. First, I would like to point out that I have an amazing medical provider. She is well-versed with disability and pointed me in the right direction. She gave me the employment development department (EDD) website information,[12] and told me exactly what I needed to do after submitting that information in order for her to complete the application.

If you don't live in California, feel free to skip ahead. This is literally a walk-through of the State Disability Insurance (SDI) process.

1. When you submit all the documentation online, which is pretty straightforward, you will get a receipt or "R" number. This is what you need to send your provider in order for them to submit their documentation.

2. At some point, EDD will send you a message through the website with the subject line "Claim for continued benefits." You will need to click on this to receive your payments.

3. Click into the hyperlink titled "Forms available to submit."

4. Click on the link titled "2500A Cert for Continued Benefits." This is the tricky part. When you are answering questions here about your disability status, you should be answering them based on your condition during the disability period. You cannot submit this form until your disability is over (or after the certification period end date they have listed), so it becomes confusing because you may no longer be disabled. However, it's important that your answers are reflective of the disability period. Therefore, you would not choose "I have

returned to work" or "I have recovered", but rather "I was unable to do my regular work because of disability throughout the certification period listed above."

The above steps are assuming you are going through SDI. Please ensure you are referencing your provider and the state for your own case, as things may change by the time you are reading this, and I am not an SDI expert.

Back to Quarantine Land

As I was nearing day 14, nothing was getting better, and by that, I mean everything was getting worse. I had dyspepsia that had me looking like I was five months pregnant ...the number of indigestion aids and antiemetics I was on was crazy. I suddenly developed a disseminated rash that looked like a gnarly allergic reaction all over my thighs. The dates are a little shaky at this point, but I do believe it was around this timeframe that I was almost through with my steroid course. In addition to that, my appetite was out of control, I was constantly feeling up and down, and of course, the steroid-induced insomnia was beginning to kick in. Luckily, I was so heavily medicated for the myriad of other symptoms that I was still sleeping most of the night and sometimes most of the day.

There's not much to say about the symptoms other than the fact that they persisted and I was unable to return to work for 40 days in total. My body was deconditioned. There are maybe three feet between my couch and the bathroom. I had to use a cane for that distance. And I felt FATIGUED after every "trip." Not only that, but the dizzy spells had kicked in, and there was no predicting when they were going to happen. I was encouraged to lie on my stomach for periods of time — imagine how much fun that is when you are constantly vomiting. This pretty much continued for the span of 40 days, but in the end, I was feeling well enough to go back to work ... At least that's what I thought. Now before we follow my return–to–work journey, you may find yourselves wondering, well what the hell did you do for 40 days ... I get you were sick, but weren't you bored? Let's answer this question next.

How to Successfully COVID As an Outpatient for 40 Days

  * Invest in some good books. I've always been a bookworm, and I have my own bookstagram page, @theunabridgedlifeofsalamacita, that I am shamelessly promoting here, but COVID reading was like no other. And when I say reading, I mostly mean audiobooks, because my arm muscles were so weak that I couldn't even lift up an electronic reader weighing less than a pound at times.

  * Watch lots of television and swap passwords with your friends. For example, my bestie also got COVID at the same time I did (no I didn't give it to her you filthy shamers, she lives across the country) and I

shared my HBO password with her because that's what friends do. And before HBO comes after me, I wasn't exceeding the available account limit, so let's put the litigation back in those pockets where it belongs. Capeesh? Okay, glad we are on the same page.

* Create bucket lists of things you plan to do after you get better. I'm afraid of heights, and I don't think anyone would ever describe me as a "thrill-seeker," but let me tell you, having your hiney glued to the couch for 40 days does stuff to you. I just wanted to feel the adrenaline pumping through my veins again. So, I made lists of activities like riding roller coasters and maybe even skydiving when I got better. Have I done any of those things? Yes! I recently went down to Universal Studios in a wheelchair and rode some roller coasters to get that adrenaline pumping. Did I skydive? No, but we can call that a dream deferred. If you are able to do some crafting, do it. Whether it's cross-stitching, quilting, lettering, putting a puzzle together — though the latter isn't really crafting — do it. This may be challenging based on your ability to stay awake, sharp, or lift a needle (no, I'm not joking) ... but if you can, power to you.

* Have lots of FaceTime and phone call sessions with your friends and family if you are able to speak without pain and if they have the time. It will truly help you feel connected emotionally.

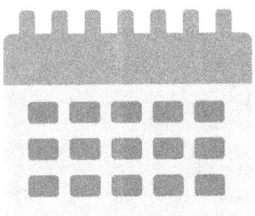

Chapter 2 : October 2021

The Body Changes

I'm not going to sit here and tell you that I've had a positive body image my whole life, because who am I kidding? We live in a culture that idolizes small waistlines, and like many, I am not immune to the messages. But also, I can tell you that I've been in therapy for over four years now, and I am happy to say I am at a point in my life where my self-worth no longer depends on my physical appearance or weight. During residency, I gained a bunch of weight and I was beginning to develop some fatty liver issues, so I was told I needed to go back to a healthier weight, and I luckily did that before COVID, and I'm happy to say I was thriving.

And then guess what happened, guys? STEROIDS, wooo!!! I was on dexamethasone which was the only thing that really made me feel better. It also claimed any appetite control or sense of satiety I had. I mean I would get these hunger chills (I think I just made up a word?) and would eat a plain bagel, then get hungry one hour later and repeat.

So naturally, I gained 20 pounds in two weeks. No, your eyes are not deceiving you: 20 pounds in 14 days. And then another 10 pounds after the initial two weeks. I developed stretch marks EVERYWHERE. Who knew you could get stretch marks above your armpits? I certainly didn't. My upper thighs looked like someone took a knife to them.

And you know what sucks about all this? If I had gotten stretch marks from a pregnancy, I would have received a tiny bundle of joy in exchange, and I would have been perfectly okay with that. But what did I get? Absolutely nothing but pain and stretch marks. I later learned that some women refer to them as beauty marks, and I have since embraced that. The medicine that was responsible for stretching my skin helped me stay alive, so yes, she's a warrior and she's embracing her beauty marks. Now, if you are going through it and reading this, the good news is, six months later as I'm writing this, they are finally starting to fade ... so don't worry, they won't always be this vivid.

In addition to these superficial changes, none of my clothing fit me anymore. I blew up overnight. So, I had to order new clothing and new work scrubs and express ship them because these changes happened so rapidly, but they were there and they were BIG, so there was no way out. No health plan could get me to lose that weight quickly, and let's be real, I was barely feeling recovered, I was not about to start any diets. So, if you are keeping a tally on expenses — that's food ordering services, underwear, bath towels, work scrubs (which are not cheap), and brand-new clothing, including shoes, because my feet grew two sizes ... I know, so rude!

The final thing I will say about body changes is that if you experience any skin conditions, it very well could be long-COVID (or COVID). I got random skin tags during COVID and on top of that, developed a specific kind of eczema on my hands during long-COVID — something I have never experienced before. Luckily, there is medication for that, and it actually helps it go away. So, if you do go through it, you aren't crazy. 'Rona's just full of unique gifts and surprises.

Back to Work Queen

Have you been keeping track with me? We said August 31st and then 40 days (including the 31st)... okay, yeah, math is hard for me too right now with the COVID fog. Luckily, I have a time-stamped selfie of my first day back to work, and that was on Saturday, October 9, 2021. Wait whaaat ... You have to work on a Saturday? Ugh, yeah, I'm an essential worker, but also, I CAN GO BACK TO WORK AND I AM OVER THE MOON ABOUT IT, because at this point I've been a couch potato for 40 days.

I was also glad my first day back was on a weekend, because sometimes those tend to be lighter than the weekdays, so I was hoping it wouldn't be too stressful. And it wasn't, which was great, because boy did I overestimate my functionality. The dizzy spells were presenting like vertigo. Any movement of my head — mostly any motion at all — made me feel like I was going to fall to the ground. My chest was very tight and I was getting runs of tachycardia as confirmed by my Apple watch. There were several instances when I had to literally stop whatever I was doing and put my head down for a few minutes or inhale some albuterol. By the end of the day, I was really scared of what this meant. I was not in any shape to perform CPR on anyone if they went down after a shot. The fog, which I didn't feel much of during my time at home, was manifesting strongly as word-finding difficulty. This is annoying to anyone really, but imagine the fear associated with this when you are a healthcare provider and your entire job is cerebral. The smallest mistake can be lethal to a patient.

I am confident in the fact that my brain fog was purely manifesting as word-finding difficulty at the time because we have several safety mechanisms in place to ensure error mitigation, but it was scary nevertheless.

I must share one particular anecdote with you to really showcase the fog that happened during my first week back at work. I was working in retail pharmacy so the final workflow before a medication is ready to be sold to the patient is that after it is filled by the technicians, the pharmacist — yours truly — scans the barcode on the vial which pulls up everything pertaining to that script on the screen, and I cross-check that with what is being dispensed.

Some things I am checking for are that it's for the right patient, it's the right medication, and visually inspecting the drug to make sure that it is in fact the right drug. After I do this, I put it in the bag, staple the patient leaflet as well as any medication guides to the bag, seal it all, then place it in a tote until the patient picks it up. Well, I did all of this, but after I was done, instead of putting it in the tote, I tossed it in the "protected information bin" that is meant for sensitive documents to be discarded.

It took a few seconds for my brain to really register that I was doing something wrong, but thank goodness it did and the medication was placed where it belonged without any repercussions to the patient or the pharmacy.

This is COVID brain. The simplest task becomes disorienting.

After my return, I was having a hard time being at work with persistent symptoms, but I knew that if I were to wait until all my symptoms vanished, then I would be out of work for a long time. Not only did I not want that for financial reasons, but this is also very frowned upon in healthcare. The unspoken rule is that as a healthcare worker, you do not get sick. And my direct supervisor made that very clear when she saw me on Monday after I returned to work.

Her first words to me were to the effect of implying that my team thought I do not care about them. I had been out for 40 days, and my team felt like I was leaving them to struggle alone.

I told her, "I'm really sorry they feel that way, but didn't they know I was sick with COVID?" My supervisor responded that it doesn't matter, they think I was enjoying my time off. I later learned that this was a complete manipulation by the individual. But at the time, I believed her, and it made me feel horrible. Here I was thinking that I'm finally semi-healthy and able to come back to work, but now I'm basically being told I'm irresponsible and a traitor for leaving my team for that long — regardless of the reason.

To make matters worse, another colleague was having a very hard time with my absence. In that colleague's defense, she had to cover many shifts while I was out. However, the fact that the first words out of her mouth to me when I came back and thanked her for the coverage was "Your apology is accepted," was wildly inappropriate.

The comments got to the point where I told her it was starting to feel like harassment and asked her to stop. I think in any job, when you use that word, people know the next step is human resources, so luckily, she stopped. But can you imagine how awful this all is? If it happened to me, chances are other people were getting similar treatment too after coming back from their illnesses. I know someone who was asked "How was your vacation?" after 10 days of quarantine. No one would say that to a cancer patient coming back from chemotherapy. So why is it okay to say that to a COVID patient? Because our perception of the disease is that it is much less severe since not everyone who gets it dies or at a minimum has to endure painful procedures and/or treatment. But guess what, many people get really sick, and some do die. And why do we need to get nasty with each other for any illness, severe or not? All that leads to is resentment and hurt feelings.

If that coworker hadn't stopped, and if I didn't need the money, I probably would have considered finding a different job, right then and there, because who wants to work at a place where they are being harassed for an illness they had no hand in acquiring? I think, in general, the lesson to be learned here is that we can do better in being understanding toward one another.

Suicide is one of the leading causes of death worldwide. With COVID, being isolated is strenuous enough for mental health. If individuals are going to be shamed once they recover, that does not seem promising for their mental health, so let's all do better, and try to be supportive. And even if we can't be supportive, we can at least choose not to say anything at all, because that will likely be more beneficial for those individuals than saying hurtful and accusatory remarks.

The Booster

Shortly after I returned to work, I freaked out about reinfection. No one really knows exactly how long antibodies last and I didn't want to take any chances, especially since my employer at the time was not taking appropriate precautions to keep us safe. So, a week after I got back and was feeling mostly normal, I took my booster shot. And then two weeks later, I was going camping with my friends, one of whom asked that we all test before we leave just to be safe. I was having some symptoms at the time, but still to my surprise, my antigen test came back positive. The timing was weird with regard to testing positive and having been boosted. Not impossible but very curious. My theory is that the negative antigen test result I had gotten prior to this test was a false negative, and I was still testing positive from the initial infection.

When I messaged my district manager — before reaching out to my provider — he said that I absolutely cannot come back to work for 10 days, regardless of what my provider said. When I spoke to my provider, she agreed that it was curious, but said that since I was having symptoms — and we did not know I was going to have long-COVID at that time — it was better to be safe and isolate. This time around was much lighter symptom-wise and my mom had come back from the east coast, so at least I had someone to help deliver food and fresh towels.

When I went back to work, the first thing my direct supervisor greeted me with, before I even entered the pharmacy was, "You need to be careful, because we can't have you keep going down like this." I don't know about you, but I find that to be just a very indelicate thing to say to someone, because it's not like I was opening the FedEx box with COVID tests and licking it. In fact, she herself later reprimanded me when I asked a patient who refused to wear a mask to show proof of his medical exemption. She also asked me to take my mask off for a group photo, even though another individual in that photo was not vaccinated at the time, so you see how inappropriate her statement was since her actions had done nothing to protect her employees from actually getting COVID. I'm not sharing this story to insult her. I'm sharing this story because I know it's not unique. In fact, I know of several people that were either pressured not to test by their employers or made to feel like garbage for being sick, and this mentality needs to stop. No one is waking up thinking, "Hmm, seems like a good day to catch some 'rona and get out of work for a few days," and yet we are treated that way.

Let's remember that this can happen to anyone. And managers, your employees will never say the things to you that you say to them if they value their jobs, so dig deep in your souls and try to find it in you to not berate your employees for getting sick, especially if you are not doing anything to protect them. Trust me, they want to be at work. With the gas prices and the economy, no one can afford to sit at home.

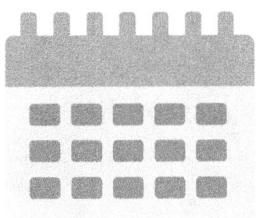

Chapter 3 : November 2021

The Bad and the Ugly

My memory is a bit hazy on all the details that happened this month. I remember my symptoms continued to worsen. I kept having ongoing diarrhea which was really interfering with my life. So bad that I will openly admit to having to wear pads at times because episodes would happen with no anticipation whatsoever. Imagine how mentally challenging that is. I'm 31 years old. Most people don't have bowel control issues at this age, and yet here I am deciding I can't leave the house without wearing a pad in case I "get the runs" all of a sudden, like how sexy is that?!

At this point, I had yet to make the connection that this was long-COVID. Around mid-November, I attempted some dietary changes to begin my journey back to a healthier weight, and I thought the new diet was the culprit, so I stopped it. But the diarrhea sure didn't. Luckily, I only had to wear pads for a week or so, which was a blessing because that is just a whole new level of crazy that nobody got time to deal with.

However, my muscle pains continued. The nausea continued. I was taking three prescription antiemetics daily with repeat dosing and still had bouts of vomiting. I know this is really disgusting, but I want you to live the picture because so many people are also going through it. Sometimes I would be talking and a small amount of vomitus would shoot up into my mouth and fall right back down my throat before I even realized what was happening. How disturbing is that? I mean the mask luckily provided a visual barrier, but really take a moment and imagine living like this, day after day after day. To top it all off, we had staffing issues at work, which is really more of a national issue, but when a pharmacy shuts down even for a day, hundreds of patients do not get their medications.

Being Overworked

I was asked to staff in a different city about an hour away several times. I was also asked to staff a double shift at my store which meant 8 a.m. to 9 p.m., with no lunch break on a few different occasions. And if you think this is sounding crazy, go do some research on working in retail pharmacy. Nevertheless, I felt pressured to do it because I had been out sick for so long, so I said yes. Well, naturally when your health is not doing great and you are putting this much stress on your body, and not being able to eat or drink, that's not going to help restore your health. My provider said it was time for me to go on disability. She thankfully recognized that I was experiencing long-COVID and that my body would never recover with those working conditions. I worked Thanksgiving and Black Friday, and have been on disability since then, with a return-to-work date of March 15, 2022, that was then pushed out to May 15, 2022, and don't worry, we will get to the why behind that shortly.

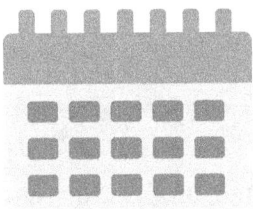

Chapter 4 : December 2021 - January 2022

Moving forward, a lot of these sections might seem scattered. Unfortunately, that's because long-COVID is very capricious and scattered. But you will definitely read a lot more on my emotions here because this is the part where it all really sets in. Where I learn to accept my long-COVID for what it is: a true disability. Where I go through the five stages of grief. Where I find out who my real friends are. Where I find out that perhaps some friendships are less than I thought they were. Where I find out about myself, my boundaries, my needs, and what I will or won't accept, even in illness. Where I find out the blessing of having had an established therapist years before this. Where I explore new hobbies that can be done on days when I am physically incapable of walking. Where I talk about all the life events and milestones that were postponed because of this. Where I talk about dating and not knowing whether I'll be able to walk that day, or if I surprise my date and show up with a cane. I'm going to talk about it all, the good, the bad, and the ugly, because otherwise, what are we doing here and how will this help anyone? So, buckle your seatbelts and get really comfy, because you are about to embark on one hell of a ride.

My first few days in December actually started off really well. My symptoms were mostly at bay and I almost found myself wondering why I was on disability. It was good for my mental health. I figured I was getting the rest my body needed, getting time to recondition my muscles to walk more than five minutes at a time, and potentially even visit my relatives if I was feeling better — something that was proving to be impossible with work.

I also realized that I would likely need to find a new job. Working for an employer that treats you poorly for getting sick is never ideal, and when they treat you like your disability is your fault ... It's time to move on. This would prove to be tricky, because I was on disability, i.e., not at my prime to interview, but I figured I would start looking because it would be a matter of weeks and I'd be back on my feet and healthy as a horse. Like I said, December started off pretty okay. I decided I would host an ugly sweater party for my coworkers and then visit my friends and family on the east coast.

Now around this time, I noticed a pattern. My PASC symptoms would disappear and resurface every three weeks. It was like clockwork. This manifested while I was traveling solo and walking across terminals in airports. During one of my layovers, I was so fatigued that I actually had to sit down for a few minutes knowing that I might full on miss my flight. My body could simply not take another step forward. So, when I got to upstate New York to visit my friend and we took a walk by the American side of the Falls, I was ecstatic at first. I hadn't been able to walk like this in a while. I made her stop a few times and had to use an inhaler, but overall, I was feeling strong.

Towards the end of the walk, I started getting very winded, but my body luckily let me power through, which was wonderful because there was not much my friend could have done to help me if I wasn't able to. But when we got back to her house, I slept for hours on end and my shins hurt so much.

This progressed when I went to Cleveland, my hometown, the next day. My family was concerned about my pain and the fact that I had to sit down after walking a few feet, but I reassured them that this was just my three-week mark. I went to visit a museum with my friend and we would walk maybe 15 feet and I would need to sit down, use an inhaler, and take a few minutes to recover. I felt really bad. Thankfully, this was one of my best friends of 10 years so I felt comfortable at least asking her to sit and wait with me.

But still, really try to picture the gravity of it all. I am someone who has no pre-existing lung— or any other — conditions. This was all because of COVID. After this hang out, I spent the remainder of my vacation at home. Very few people were using masks — I was one of the only people still wearing one, it seemed— and because I was super scared to catch a new infection, I preferred to stay home. I was also feeling very tired and fatigued.

I went back to California and crap hit the fan. I was starting to feel very tired very frequently. I thought it was side effects from the new medication I was on; however, the medication was stopped, and nothing really changed. My symptoms went from every three weeks to every three days to almost every day. I got this calf tightness that worsened with any movement, and I'm still dealing with that today. If I am able to walk long enough without respiratory issues, my calf tightens up and I start limping a little. The chills that never went away were increasing in severity. I was doing a virtual paint night with a friend — at home and fully masked— and toward the end, the chills got so bad they were hindering my ability to paint.

When something like this happens and I'm with someone outside of my family, I go through many emotions. Do I tell the person what's going on, or will that weird them out? You might be reading this and thinking why would that weird them out, but you have no idea how awkward people can get when I share.

Some people don't say anything and that, to me, is literally the worst response because it makes me wonder "Do you not care that I'm suffering?" Other people get squirrely and awkward but at least say something to acknowledge it like, "I'm sorry that's happening" or "That sucks." And of course, there are always the champions of "Don't worry it'll be fine" and that is how you really piss off Salam, because no, sir, you do not in fact know that it will be fine. If my provider cannot provide me with a guarantee of it being fine, then no one else can. But I digress.

My point is there are so many uncomfortably vulnerable feelings that happen when these symptoms come up. It is so much easier to close yourself off from the rest of the world until you are better, even though you may not know when or if better will ever come. That's why it is very important for acquaintances of long-haulers to check in on them regularly and reassure them that you want to spend time with them and are happy to accommodate their limitations— assuming of course that this is true.

This disease is very isolating. You seem like you are semi-okay, but in actuality, you are very restricted. You may not have lost functionality, but certain health limitations may come up every now and then, and this is the problem. No one knows or can predict when these limitations will come up and that is very stressful because you don't know what you are supposed to acclimate to.

You can only make plans with friends if they are fully aware that you may have to cancel at the last minute because your health literally can change that much and that quickly. If you love to go hiking like me, perhaps you are able to at first, but all of a sudden, your health declines and now you can't. The primary activity that you do to help get yourself out of a funk is now taken away from you and that's really hard. You may even lose friendships over this. If you met your group of friends through mutual hobbies, it will be very difficult to hang out if your activities are now limited. Hopefully, this doesn't completely rupture a friendship, but it can certainly present challenges because your friends care about you, but they may not feel inclined to alter their lifestyles to align with yours, and unfortunately, that's probably most people.

So, if you are going through it, I hear you, and I get it, and I'm sorry. If you know someone who is, try and be there for them. Even if it's just once a month, even if it means drinking tea and sitting with them instead of going rock climbing like you wanted... be there for them. It may only be one hour of your life, but to the patient, it means the world, because this is now all of their life.

Continued Decline

In the following few weeks, my health continued to decline. So much so that I felt like I was back in COVID. I can't tell you how many antigen tests and NAATs[2] I did that all came back negative. On days when

---

2. Nucleic Acid Amplification Test.

I was feeling semi-okay, I didn't trust myself to go to a grocery store or walk outside alone because the deterioration would happen so fast. Even taking care of regular chores became difficult.

I was filled with embarrassment, fear, and guilt. Embarrassment because I couldn't take care of my normal needs. If I had the energy to cook, I didn't have the energy to wash the dishes. I certainly didn't have the energy to take out the trash, because for months after COVID, just lifting a bag into the communal dumpster would render my arms sore. My cat's litter box was not being cleaned every day. And I didn't have the energy to clean my bathrooms, dust, etc. I luckily have a robot vacuum, but even having to clear the floor from cat toys and clothes was at times too challenging. I bought a bunch of plastic plates, cups, and utensils, which added to the charges but at least allowed me to not live in the fear of getting a bug infestation with the dirty dishes.

I finally mustered up the courage to ask my mom if she would be willing to help me clean my toilet or take out the trash if I needed that. This was probably the hardest and most painful thing I have ever had to do in my life, which is weird because I'm a straight shooter that usually needs to tone down the bluntness (I'm sure you can tell from this book). For some reason, though, being that vulnerable and asking my mom to take care of my most primal needs was different. Of course, my mom being the sweet angel that she is said "of course" and that I should ask her anytime. She reassured me that I should never feel embarrassed to ask, and if she was truly busy or tired that day — my biggest fear behind asking her and making her feel pressured to help me — she would just come over the next day. When I got that response, I cried.

Being this disabled is very humbling. I mentioned why I was embarrassed, but let's talk about fear and guilt. When you are a healthy adult, you probably don't think about your gradual health decline every day. We all know it's inevitable, but we don't want to ruin the party, so we delay thinking about it. It's scary to think about how much we could depend on others. Personally, I am very independent in general, partly personality and partly due to life circumstances. When you move away from family for school and are confronted by the unkind reality of many people, you learn to not rely on anyone because many people will say they will be there for you but somehow always have something come up if you actually need them, even if they know you have no family or significant other in town. So, the thought of being sick becomes terrifying.

I live in the same town as my parents now, but when I got COVID, they were both out of the state and for pressing reasons. Again, all very terrifying. You fear that you will be a burden if you ask, and even more, you fear that you will be refused help when you are at your weakest. That is a pain that no words can describe. You become fearful that you are being a burden that will ultimately lead your family to detach or get drained from looking after you. I had many days when I feared what my decline in health would lead to in the long run.

Would burdening my mom with carrying out my trash and cleaning my bathroom all become too much? Were my parents secretly wishing I would move back in with them and make their lives easier? That is a level of independence I hope I never have to forfeit, but these are the thoughts that were going on in my head and still continue to on days when my health takes a step backwards. But this allowed me to empathize with other disabled individuals as well as my grandparents. I have a friend on Bookstagram who is dealing with chronic pain and disability in her early 20s, and she talks a lot about living by herself and how it actually helps out her family financially, but also how important this level of autonomy is for her mental health. I get that now.

My grandmas, both strong and loving Mediterranean women, show their love through food. Unfortunately, both are getting older, to the point where cooking an elaborate or even simple Syrian meal actually gives them back pain and arm pain because of all the needed prep work. And yet the daily debacles that happen any time we visit them— one lives in Florida and the other lives in Ohio— are comical. They refuse to let anyone assist them at all costs. I used to think they were being stubborn and impractical (sorry grandmas, I love you!) but now I get it.

This is literally all they have left to feel like their

past powerful selves. One of them always needs a walker to ambulate and the other refuses to use a walking aid and in turn, spends lots of time on the couch or in bed. So, cooking for them is not just an act of love; it's a marker of autonomy and independence, and it is VERY hard to let that go. You are essentially admitting that you are less of a human. Not in worth or value, but certainly in physical ability, and who wants to be that weak and vulnerable? No one.

As hard as it is for me, I actually do give in on days when I'm this tired, and by days, I mean prolonged stretches that don't allow me air to breathe and do things like clean the restroom or meal prep. I am so grateful for the help I get, and I do my best to let my mom know how much I appreciate her. But I still feel guilty. I always wonder if her job would be easier if I moved in with her and my dad. But I know how detrimental that would be to my autonomy and mental health. Not because there is anything wrong with my family or that living arrangement — after all, they have a spare bedroom with a bed in it — but it would make me feel like I've taken so many steps back at 31, an age where many are starting families of their own. Therefore, I choose to accept her help and be grateful, in hopes that I never become a full-on burden to her.

If your health condition is much worse and you have had to make changes to your living arrangement or do feel this way, I will share something my therapist told me that helped. In any kind of close relationship, you will inevitably be a burden on the person, and they will be a burden on you, because that is the nature of close relationships and that is okay.

This was a big pill for me to swallow but it's been very helpful, so remember that. And if you are reading this and you are the caregiver, thank you. Sometimes the person you are looking after may be so exhausted physically and emotionally that they may forget to thank you, or they may be so irritable from it all that they come off as ungrateful even if they don't mean to be. To that, I say thank you. You are keeping this person's life going and for that you deserve the world.

Gratitude

I've talked a lot about my mom physically being there for me, but let's talk about her and my dad some more. As you know by now, up to this point, I've been on disability. This translates into 50% of my regular paycheck. Now at first, this was fine, but soon I started to panic because I couldn't stop my private student loan payments for more than three months, and I didn't want to use that option right away. I was also relying on delivery services. Something I still struggle with is giving my parents, neighbors, or any friends who ask, a grocery list. I'm very specific. I want a certain brand and flavor of yogurt, for example, and feel very high-maintenance asking for that. I also have random needs, sometimes, at strange hours of the day. For example, I ran out of cough syrup and really needed some at 11 pm. I wasn't going to call up my parents for that, but luckily there are plenty of DoorDashers in my area who are happy to help. But again, this leads to more and more expenses.

This is all in addition to the many medical expenses. So, my parents graciously offered to pay for my groceries and gas. Of course, I refused; however, what I did accept is sometimes they would go grocery shopping and "happen to pick up a salmon filet or some heirloom tomatoes for me" or "bought some extra toilet paper and paper towels from Costco and thought you might need some." These obvious yet subtle gestures of love that translate into decreased financial costs for me mean the world. I know I'm lucky that my parents have the means to help me. I'm still embarrassed and a little guilty for needing and accepting this assistance, but I couldn't survive well without it.

If you have someone in your life who is truly offering to help, no strings attached, try to let them help. You won't help your health improve by not eating any protein because you are trying to cut costs. Believe me, I know how hard this is, but accepting it can really help you. And to be completely honest, I did cave and fill my car with gas from them once, but this was before the prices skyrocketed, so I feel a little better about that.

In the next section, you will read about my travels to seek a higher level of care. I relied fully on my dad's frequent flyer miles to book several tickets to and from home. I relied fully on his and my mom's financial assistance to rent a car so I could go to the doctors' appointments. I very much needed to have my mom travel with me because I can't always walk unassisted, which used up time, her most valuable real estate.

I also accepted their payment for a trip to Universal Studios, something I could never afford on my own with my current finances. This last year has been strenuous to say the least, and I knew that a day at Universal Studios would do wonders for my mood (remember the adrenaline rush we talked about), so I accepted their help. Of course, naturally, as you will read about shortly, I came back with ... A BRAND NEW COVID INFECTION from Universal Studios, but that one's on me. Still did wonders for my mood and I think everyone deserves that after being in this never-ending pandemic.

Our society teaches us that being disabled means suffering. Well, here's a newsflash, if you are disabled, you are already suffering, there's no need to pile on and make it worse. If you do have assistance of any kind, accept it. You deserve it and are worthy of it.

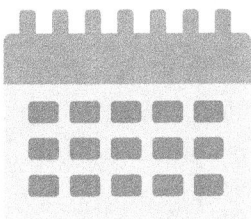

Chapter 5 : February 2022

Thoughts

February has probably been the toughest month emotionally. I'll start with an excerpt from my diary :

What has my life been reduced to? I am now attempting to choose student loan refinance options based on the opportunity to be discharged if I have a permanent disability. I am 31 years old. People are planning on advancing their careers, starting families, and going on vacations at this age. Meanwhile, yours truly is realizing that her whole life might have been upended because of COVID-19. I'm feeling anger and rage. I'm feeling resentment. And all those feelings are directed at the person who decided not to enforce "wearing masks" i.e., covering your nose at work. Because maybe, just maybe, I wouldn't be in this situation right now if he had done that. I'm also feeling humbled. I can be as angry and pissed off as I want to be, but none of that will change my reality.

I am also feeling helpless and vulnerable. I hate

that I have to text my friends to check on me. But I have to remind myself that while I have all the time in the world on my hands, they are all living their lives with their own ups and downs, and unfortunately as adults that means they won't remember my long–COVID or think to check in because who can imagine that a healthy 31–year–old would be going through all this. Several of my friends got COVID during this time period and it hit them hard, but most haven't had any lingering symptoms, so I can see how hard it would be for them to empathize or realize what I'm going through. I also hate that I'm feeling a little resentful. It's not that I'm not happy that they recovered. I'm just angry that I didn't. Why me? And I know this is all part of the stages of grief. I realize that I'm grieving my own health while I'm alive because I don't know what's left of it. This all just sucks.

I feel a deep gratitude for my mom. The woman has never invalidated a single symptom or emotion since this curse that is COVID has been thrust into my life. The single person who has literally been there for me through it all. She's tolerated MANY emotions and believe me there have been many.

I told my mom she is allowed to complain and vent in front of me. I recognized that as my mom she is grieving her daughter's health too and that is probably very hard for her. She's been holding it together for me. I told her it's okay for her not to. She's allowed to talk to me about her fears over my health and where it's at and where it hasn't gotten. It won't make my situation any worse. This brought us closer. We are very different. I confront things head on, she is a lot more passive and gentle. I've learned that she needs to tell herself that things aren't always what they are to cope. I will give her space to do that because she is also grieving. I love that we can be this vulnerable and open with each other despite our vastly different communication styles and personalities.

I just want this hell to end. It's like no one believes I'm sick or seems to care because I don't have cancer and didn't undergo surgery so no one cares enough to send me a card or flowers or acknowledge me in any way — except for my mom because she's the greatest, but I want others to care about me too. So many people I thought were friends haven't even responded to texts or posts about my health, yet they have no problem responding when I comment on their latest adventures in life. Do they think they will accidentally catch the "rona" if they show me some care, or do they really just not give a fuck? I don't know, but I sure know not to go out of my way for them if they can't even be bothered to respond to a text. It just sucks, and it's isolating, and it's not fair. I just want it to end already.

I feel really guilty about how I treated her. I don't know why I never found two hours to drive down and visit her during hospice. She was such a close friend and I cared so much about her. And now she's gone and I will never get a chance for a redo. I wish I had the foresight back then to know how much a visit would have meant to her. I hate myself right now for being so self-absorbed. It would have been half a day out of my entire life. Now I know what a selfish asshole I was. I'm glad I at least got to have one final birthday lunch with her. I hope she's in a better place now surrounded with lots of angels and peace.

* For reference my friend was diagnosed with cancer during pharmacy school and she persevered through it all. She became an angel shortly before we graduated.

Dating

February was a rough month. All my emotions were converging and not in a good way. I was back on dating apps and I was having to talk to guys about my long-COVID, which sucked. On the one hand, it was great because I'm looking for a serious relationship, so mentioning it helped me weed some people out very quickly. On the other hand, there were some awesome guys, but I didn't necessarily want to be this vulnerable with them because I didn't really know any of them yet. The problem is, long-COVID doesn't care, and if I was going to make plans to meet someone a week from today, for example, I had no way of predicting whether I would be experiencing dizzy spells that day, having shortness of breath, or be feeling fine and dandy. So, what do I do? I wasn't going to put a pin in dating any longer. I did that for a few months to wait until I was fully recovered, but then I realized that this may be my new normal.

No one knows exactly how "long" long-COVID is. I believe there is a lid for every pot, but I will not find my partner by sitting at home and staying off of dating apps. Since I couldn't really leave home, I knew I had to Tinder and Bumble away. One of the guys I was talking to was very nice, but I could tell it was not going to work out for other reasons, so meeting up in real life never became an issue.

It was interesting however, to see how my perspective was being shifted by long-COVID. This guy was a runner and made it a point to talk about how he enjoyed running eight miles every day and how he was going to get me to like running (unrelated to COVID). Now, this was all during a FaceTime date and it was really getting on my last nerve because I was over here telling this person that I was happy I'd been able to walk for about 15 minutes every day for the last maybe four days, and he was going on and on about his daily eight-mile runs.

I bring this up to showcase the complexity of dating for people going through long-COVID, especially those who led a fairly active life pre-COVID. You are being told that you will get back to baseline, so you try and find someone with similar interests. But you are not at baseline. So, you may get irritated and feel like the other person is being insensitive to your condition. At the same time, in my case at least, I didn't want to date people that had no interest in the outdoors or exercising, because that's what I like to do for fun and that's where I plan to be if and when my health recovers. It is the ultimate catch-22. Like I said, luckily with this guy, there were other reasons why I knew it wouldn't work out, so I didn't have to feel bad about my long-COVID getting in the way of a potential relationship, but it definitely gave me something to think about.

Now this second guy I matched with seemed nice and he was very empathetic about everything I was going through. Our timing was working out very well because I was busy dealing with my health and he had some things going on, so it seemed perfect. But the closer we got to actually meeting up, the more panicked I became, because crap hit the fan (again) halfway through February. On Valentine's Day, I spent a very romantic evening in the emergency department where I was diagnosed with pleuritis, also known as pleurisy.[13,14] In a nutshell, this is an inflammation of the membranes surrounding the lungs, resulting in lots of pain with breathing or any kind of movement, including talking.

A Quick Detour to the Emergency Room

Before we find out who gets the rose, let's take a quick detour from dating and segue back to the pleuritis. Around the end of January or early February, I was slowly able to walk again. I was still having dizzy spells and my knees would buckle up, but the episodes were less severe. Every day I would go to my parent's house and coerce my mom into walking a short distance with me. I didn't trust myself to walk alone. This walk which should take ~5-10 minutes would take me 15-20 minutes depending on the day. This also included stopping to use my inhaler, holding on to her as I got dizzy, and sitting down altogether because my legs could no longer support me. This happened every day, every time — no exaggeration whatsoever. But I wanted to keep challenging my body. My provider made it very clear that I would not be hindering my recovery in any way by doing this, so I wanted to see if walking a little bit every day would somehow prevent me from going deep in the trenches when the symptoms got worse. I always did this while wearing a pulse oximeter, and would check my blood pressure before and after.

Part of my long-COVID is rapid changes in my vitals for no apparent reason. In addition, when I walked outside or if I tried to walk on the treadmill, my heart muscle would often hurt, and this was usually accompanied by a drop in my oxygen saturation to 94%; however, this was usually transient, so I wasn't super concerned. Now the blood pressure part is really weird for me. Out of the blue, I would get tired (and this still happens) and my blood pressure would drop to 96/58 mmHg and my heart rate would also drop to 40 beats per minute. This meant I'd have to sit down or lie down immediately because I would feel like all the energy was zapped out of my system. And sometimes my blood pressure would be normal but my heart rate would spike to 111 beats per minute at rest, for no apparent reason. All these changes back-to-back had me feeling off balance, and they are a big part of why I didn't trust myself to walk anywhere alone, but I knew I had to keep going to rebuild my stamina. I did these walks with my mom, or some days with my next-door neighbor. When I was feeling off balance, I would use my cat's stroller — yes, Luna is a queen and she has a stroller — for balance, similar to that provided by a walker. This really helped me to drag my legs when it was difficult to bend my knees and walk.

The week before Valentine's Day, it became more and more difficult. I would have to sit down abruptly on the ground and have to take very deep breaths. My chest was in pain. I started to feel like I was getting really short of breath. And at night I couldn't lie down. It was PAINFUL. It felt like my chest was on fire and I couldn't breathe. This was not conducive to the insomnia that I had been experiencing for just over a month. So now instead of falling asleep at 12 a.m. (my normal is 9:30 pm, don't judge), I couldn't sleep from the pain until 2 a.m. each day.

In addition, I was feeling strange mood shifts at night. I was getting intrusive thoughts like I'd never experienced before. I felt myself getting very paranoid and having strange mood shifts. No matter how positive the day was, once night fell, it felt like my brain was trying to find something negative to fixate on and make me sad. It felt like it had to do with COVID, but I didn't want to believe it because it seemed too far-fetched. I felt like I was crazy. I would later confirm with a provider that all this may in fact be strongly caused by the virus.

Now, I live in Humboldt County, California. We are such a beautiful place to live in and visit especially if you love the outdoors, but unfortunately, we are very underserved medically speaking. This is important to know because when I messaged my provider on MyChart and she requested an urgent CT scan for my chest because of the chest pain and difficulty breathing, the earliest appointment was two weeks out. I even checked a slightly larger city that was a three-hour drive away, and they were also at capacity with no sooner appointments.

My provider told me that if my breathing kept worsening, I should go to the emergency department. I thought I could tough it out, but by the evening of Valentine's Day, I could not breathe very well. It was very strange because my oxygenation wasn't low, but I would have to take these very deep inhalations every few minutes to feel like I could breathe, and I was in pain. I was visiting my parents that evening and they suggested that I wait until the morning because that's when the emergency department is typically emptier, and also, so that I don't get home late at night. Of course, my parents are the kindest people and were begging me to come back to their place after dinner, but they know how stubborn their daughter is and that I'd want to go home to my cat, hence their gentle nudging toward the morning visit. But my breathing kept getting harder and more and more painful, so I decided to go to the ER because I wasn't going to fall asleep before 2 a.m. anyway, so no matter the duration of the wait, I would be okay.

The ER visit was transformative for me. I finally decided to open up about my story. Believe it or not, I am very uncomfortable being vulnerable. But I was also tired of feeling so isolated. And tired of seeing people act like COVID is not a big deal. Because it probably wasn't a big deal for them, but not everyone gets to recover as quickly, and all stories need to be heard. I decided to move forward and share my "Long-Hauler Chronicles," even though I was scared of being criticized and rejected. I started with an introductory poem about my Valentine's Day from the ER. I shared this on my blog, Facebook, LinkedIn, Instagram, and Twitter. I was overwhelmed by the responses.

So many people sent the kindest messages, and to that, I say thank you. You made a difference in my life. I was feeling very alone and isolated, and knowing that you care made a really big difference. When you are gradually becoming disabled, whether it's temporary or permanent, your health is deteriorating alone. You are literally becoming more and more reliant on other people, so it matters to know that other people will be there, or at least care, if you need them. This is why reaching out, or liking a status update pertaining to health, or any other form of actively showing the person you are thinking about them makes such a big difference in that person's life. So again, thank you to everyone who showed me they care.

After posting that Valentine ER post, I decided to create an Instagram account called @longhaulerchronicles where I post about the day-to-day things. For example, I really needed a new jewelry box, but finances were tight and I knew I was going to be accruing more medical expenses, so I used a Styrofoam board and wooden skewers to DIY a makeshift necklace holder. Another post was on a day when I woke up feeling okay, decided to do the dishes, and all of a sudden, noticed big pools of sweat just dripping from my forehead into the sink, accompanied by chills. The plans for the day quickly changed into me laying down in bed with some snacks, water, and a small diamond paint canvas. This is one of the few hobbies I can do in bed — of course, the chills make it difficult, but when they dissipate, I can pick it up again. I use the 8x11-inch canvases, so they fit on a lightweight clipboard, and I usually listen to an audiobook or have TV on in the background. There are many great audio services that can get you a large selection of audiobooks for under $10 a month. I use Scribd for example.

I don't believe I shared all the details from the rest of that day on that long-hauler post, but I will tell you, it was bad. My mom was actually not feeling too great either, but she was well enough to toss the ingredients I ordered from DoorDash into my air fryer for me because she knew I was way too weak to walk or prepare any kind of food for myself that day.

In addition to these daily tidbits of my life, I developed a weekly post, addressing some emotion or aspect of long-COVID. This is what I share on all my social media platforms (except for Twitter and TikTok — sorry). I know that many people don't read the text in photos, so I made sure to bullet point the main concepts and then delve into the details for those who wanted to read the actual blog post.

I am saddened to say I haven't been able to post every week. Some weeks the symptoms are bad and they are persistent. But I hope my followers can understand that the nature of this beast is that it's fickle, and sometimes I am too tired and unable to post. This should also help people empathize with why so many long-haulers unfortunately have had to miss days of work or go on disability, because this is how it goes.

Back to the ER, though. Because the hospitals were so saturated, I was given the option to wait in my car after triage. Essentially, I went into a side room where they did a quick EKG, got my vitals, and drew some blood tests and then they sent me to my car. Then they called me to come in for the CT of my lungs, then they sent me back to my car again until there was finally a bed available for me.

To be honest, I didn't mind this at all because I listened to a full Colleen Hoover audiobook from start to finish — that's how busy the ER was. But in the meantime, I was checking my results live as they were becoming available through the patient portal and I saw that my d-dimer was a bit elevated. I took this to mean I may have a pulmonary embolism or a clot in my lungs and was surprisingly happy because I figured "well at least I would know what the cause of this incessant lung pain and difficulty breathing is" and it's treatable. At the time I thought to myself "I'm obese, I have not been moving at all because I'm unable to, COVID may increase risk of clots, and I'm on hormonal birth control which also increases risk for clots, so it makes sense."

It ended up not being a pulmonary embolism, which in hindsight, I am grateful for. Turns out, it was pleuritis, and there is not much that can be done to resolve it. Some medications were encouraged to help alleviate the pain, but the only way to get rid of it is to treat the underlying cause, which is COVID, or in my case, long-COVID.

I have been living with this wonderful pleuritis since that night and it's honestly been one of the most strenuous symptoms to deal with because it impacts my daily activities in so many ways. Even though my oxygenation isn't affected, I feel so short of breath when I'm walking, talking, laughing, breathing, and especially when I'm lying down, so imagine how hard it is to sleep. Most nights I end up either propping up three couch cushions or lying on my belly in order to minimize the pain and be able to sleep.

This of course is with open-mouthed breathing. Because I feel so winded, I can't walk more than a few steps without having to sit down. And naturally, my muscles get even more deconditioned and it just gets harder and harder to rebuild my stamina with the ongoing symptoms. The pain medications and inhaler helped a little bit, but they weren't life-changing. What did give me hope was the ER physician. He listened to me and validated my symptoms. He kept reassuring me that this was not in my head. He told me that they, meaning the medical providers, were seeing this all the time with COVID survivors: people who are young and healthy before COVID that end up like me on disability. He told me that he's seen a lot of people recover around the six-month mark, but for some, it takes longer. He told me that my symptoms are actually within the normal scope of long-COVID and that he had faith that I would recover from all my symptoms, he just can't tell me when.

I remember tearing up when he said that and I was so embarrassed, but it was the first glimmer of hope I'd seen in a long time. I also realized that I was not alone in feeling like it was in my head. The way the symptoms are so on and off really makes you question your sanity, so having a medical professional who regularly treats patients like me confirm how normal my experience was, made me feel better. I was also encouraged that I would be able to go to work because I felt so much anguish in being a fairly fresh graduate that should be on the front line with the said provider, but instead, I'm on disability. Overall, I left the ER feeling very hopeful for what the future holds. This was very close to my return-to-work date; however, due to the new pleuritis diagnosis, my provider extended my disability leave until mid-May.

The Cleveland Clinic

Around this time, my friend who lives in Cleveland told me that the Cleveland Clinic has a long-COVID recovery clinic. I decided to search and see if there was something like this where I lived or in other places in Northern California. I figured I'm on disability and I thankfully have insurance, so this would be the time to seek treatment. I knew this might lead to some medical costs, but I also saw how heavily the disease was impacting my life. While outsiders may not see it like a serious, potentially terminal illness — and dear God I hope it's not — it definitely has a similar impact because I am literally having to put everything on hold, and I am getting worse and worse every day. If one symptom improves, a new symptom comes up.

I think around that time is when I actually registered how serious my own situation was. It turned out that my area did not have any such resources. I looked at one of the large medical centers in Northern California and that institution's website was a little misleading. It had information presented in a way that insinuates a long-hauler clinic, but when I called them, I found out they did not actually have that service. Instead, you had to meet very stringent criteria and then you would be transferred to a pulmonologist and different specialists from there. This seemed a bit too tedious. So, I called the Cleveland Clinic. I also felt very comfortable doing this because I actually did my post-graduate residency training at one of the Cleveland Clinic hospitals and I am originally from Cleveland, Ohio, so it didn't feel as intimidating. My grandma and uncle live in Cleveland, so I also knew I could stay with them for free, whereas anywhere else, I'd have to pay for lodging, and I didn't have that kind of money.

I was blown away by the ease of scheduling an appointment. I was also blown away that my insurance considered the clinic "in-network," meaning my medical bills would not be exorbitantly more expensive than if I were to be seen in my current city. This is one of many reasons why I will be tooting the Cleveland Clinic's horn for a little bit, and no they are not paying me to say this. The fact that the Clinic is contracted with so many insurance providers and has a national physician — for those like myself who are traveling to be treated — is truly exceptional. It provides people with hope. Especially people like myself who need a higher level of care and expertise, and who at times feel trapped because they live in very rural areas that do not offer such care. Thank you.

Back to California

About a week after I left the ER, the pleuritis started to resolve and oh man was I feeling better. It was so mind-boggling how unpredictable and spontaneous the improvements and deteriorations were.

I noticed it one night when I was laying down to sleep and my pain level went from a 100% to maybe a

40%. I remember telling my parents the next day it was a lot less pain, mostly discomfort, and that was an improvement.

Within a few days, I was feeling much better. One day, I was feeling so good that I was able to take a 20-minute walk with my mom again. The next day, I pushed my limits and did some cleaning around the house. My energy would wane by the afternoon, but it was still mostly there. I couldn't believe it. On day three, I was over the moon. I packaged all the books I was selling for a side hustle and shipped them out.

This has been one of the best gifts of long-COVID. Your good days are so limited that you really become a time-management machine. You don't know how many you will get, so you knock off everything you need to do as efficiently as you can.

But here's the kicker: the good days kept coming. A walk around my neighborhood that usually takes 50 minutes only took me 35 minutes. This was HUGE. I thought I was over the hump and clearly on the path to recovery. So much so that I was actually considering canceling my appointment with the Cleveland Clinic — thank God I didn't. I decided that I didn't want to take any chances, and if nothing else, it would be a nice getaway to see my family and friends in Cleveland.

Back to Dating

Let's go back to the gentleman suitor at the beginning of February. Before I started to feel better, I wasn't sure what to do. Do I bring a cane on the date in case I get dizzy? We are both outdoorsy people — at least I was before long-COVID — so we were talking about a small hike or something fun outdoors. As much as I wanted to do that, I was terrified about what my health would do. I was also unsure if I should keep talking to him. I felt like I was somehow deceiving him, because what if I don't get better? This is a very different headspace than getting sick after you're in an established relationship with someone. This is someone you are meeting for the first time, and they don't have a reason to change their life for you. After all, if you enjoy hiking every weekend, how happy are you going to be in a relationship with someone who can't share your main hobby with you? It was very mentally challenging.

I asked my close friends and they all said, "If he doesn't like you with the cane, then he doesn't deserve you." My mom said something similar. But I still wasn't convinced, because honestly, it took me months to mentally accept walking with a cane. It's not that I am ashamed of it or feel that I am less worthy because of it. It's just an adaptation...but, at that time it felt like springing that on someone who doesn't know me was kind of unfair.

On the one hand, if his face showed visible

surprise, it would make me feel bad. And on the other hand, if he didn't, it just felt like a lot of pressure to put on a first date when none of my pictures reflected that (because my health at the time I set up my profile was okay). The more I thought about it, the more it started to feel like a test. I went from not wanting to have a cane to thinking "Maybe I should, because if it turns him off, does that mean that if I get sick down the line he will bolt and not be supportive?" I knew this thinking was flawed, because "testing" someone is never a healthy way to start a relationship, but that's how I was feeling.

So, what did Salam do? She set up an appointment with her therapist.

My therapist helped me recognize that a first date should be fun and I should set myself up for success. Not in an "I should be healthy or no one will like me" type of way, but rather in an "I should be having fun and engaging in activities that allow me to be my true self" type of way.

We talked about how taking a walk or a hike and worrying about getting a dizzy spell or getting winded after five minutes would not be fun for me. Therefore, I would not be setting myself up for success to see if I honestly enjoyed the company of this person. We talked about how someone's first facial expression when they see the cane is not necessarily an accurate indicator of how caring and reliable, they would be in an actual relationship. We talked about how I could decide to go on a hike with a cane and that could lead to a positive or negative relationship down the road, and that could also happen if I decided to meet this guy at a coffee shop. Ultimately, there are many factors that contribute to whether one date becomes two, or more, and adding undue physical stress by forcibly exerting myself was completely unnecessary.

I decided when the time came, I would propose a more relaxed activity like grabbing coffee. Except I suddenly got better and I was super confident that all the cane business was behind me. Now before you start rooting for a burgeoning romance, I'm going to tell you that we never met and nothing happened and that's okay. The gentleman had a few pre-planned trips of his own and then I traveled to Cleveland to get treated so things naturally fizzled out.

The good news is that I learned a lot about myself and dating through this disability. It's HARD. You are forced to be vulnerable and open at a much earlier stage than anyone ever really wants to be when they are first getting to know someone. There's no right or wrong answer on whom you should pursue because you have no idea how your disability will limit you and how long it will last. What I did decide for myself is that if my disability persists, even if I think someone might have an issue with it or assume that they will see it as a burden, I won't be the one to make that decision for them because they may not perceive it that way. It is so hard for some of us, or at least me, to accept that what we perceive as a burden may not be that way for someone else, or maybe it is but we are still worth it for them.

My biggest advice if you are dating in this rough and tumble long-COVID stage is don't push away other people solely because you think they won't be able to handle it with you. People will surprise you. I didn't even meet this guy in person, but I opened up to him a little about my disability and he seemed incredibly kind and understanding. That won't be everyone, but you'll never know if you never try. And if you put a pin in dating while you are going through this, that is also okay. No one can tell you what is right or wrong for you. There are so many emotions that you are going through, and if dating is an added stressor and you feel better pausing it altogether, then you have every right to.

I will end the chapter on dating with this final anecdote. When I went to Universal Studios, I was in a wheelchair. I saw a recently wedded couple — per their custom-design shirts — and they looked to be my age, early thirties, and the wife was in a wheelchair being pushed by her husband. This gave me all the hope in the world. It reaffirmed what my friends always tell me: wheelchair or not, disability or not, there will always be good guys and good girls out there that will not fixate on this one attribute and write me off completely because of it. Do I hope to need ambulatory aids forever? No, for many many reasons. But I know that if I do need them, I will find a guy who loves me regardless.

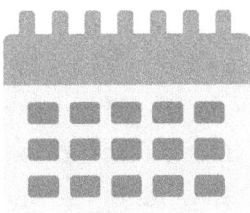

Chapter 6 : March 2022

Dr. Sullivan

On March 2, 2022, I woke up in Cleveland, Ohio feeling excited and nervous. I'm a pretty high-strung person and when I'm nervous my brain tends to make really big leaps into worst-case scenarios. My biggest fear was that I had traveled over 2,000 miles to be seen by a provider that was going to dismiss my symptoms and spend 10 minutes with me instead of the allotted 60 minutes. I was getting pissed just thinking about it.

Luckily, my sweet, even-tempered mom told me to calm the heck down in so many words because I was going to see a professional at the number two hospital in the world for specialty care. So, I tried. When I went there, I showed up with a list of my 41 PASC symptoms and I was ready to tell him all about it.

We got there 30 minutes early—type-A personality here — and I was amazed that they let us in right away. Now this obviously would not have been possible if there was a patient right before me, but still, my experience with providers in the past is that you wait at least 10-30 minutes after your appointment time, if not more. I was impressed. When Dr. Sullivan came in, he immediately filled the exam room with an air of calmness. He took time to introduce himself and never made me feel like he was hard-pressed to get out and see the remainder of his patients. We went through all 41 symptoms in-depth. He interjected where appropriate to ask questions and provide me with information. For example, when I talked about the fog and the increasing forgetfulness that was terrifying me, he provided two anecdotes about famous people he knew that had long and successful careers. They were fearful of losing their jobs because their employers could not fathom what it means that by 1 pm their brains could no longer function properly. All their tests and values came back normal, so what could possibly be wrong? But this in fact is the curse that is long-COVID, and this is why it's hard to grasp for people who are not experiencing it.

I cannot describe how much solace his words provided me with. He made me feel seen and heard. In a world where I can see the astonishment on everyone else's faces when I describe any of my symptoms, he made me feel normal. He was also very honest. He told me that overall, I am on the uptrend, and he was confident that I would be able to return to work by mid-May — though no guarantees were made because no one can say with 100% certainty.

He also made it very clear that if my symptoms were to decline again — remember I was on an upswing — that this is normal. Until the symptoms are all gone, I would likely continue to experience waxes and wanes and that's all part of it. He gave me the option to either enroll in the reCOVer Clinic[15]— the designated long-hauler clinic— or to have him order any labs and tests and refer me to the necessary specialists. He explained that the services they were going to provide me with were very similar to what he had to offer, except with a potentially longer timeline due to demand volume. Because I was traveling, we decided that having him be my primary care provider was the best plan for me.

If you are reading this and are super impressed that we had all these discussions during that one meeting, you should be. We all know what an ideal provider is supposed to do: listen to the patient, discuss treatment options with them, and make sure the patient is part of the decision-making process, but in reality, how often does that happen?

I will say I'm fortunate that my provider in Humboldt is also like this, but I've certainly had providers that made it feel like they were doing me a favor by spending five minutes with me. I recognize that healthcare requires a lot more documentation nowadays, and there are numbers that need to be met, so I don't mean this as a criticism to other providers. But when you see extraordinary care, it is important to recognize it, and that is what Dr. Sullivan provided. When you read this, Dr. Sullivan, thank you from the bottom of my heart. No matter what happens with my health, you made a significant impact on my life that day.

Testing Devices, Canes, Wheelchairs, and Empathy

We ran a few labs after the appointment and the one abnormal value was my blood sugar. It came back at 50 mg/dL, which is very low. I thought it was because I hadn't had much to eat that morning, but obviously it was worth looking into, especially because this could explain the brain fog and it was easily fixable. We discussed measuring a few random blood sugar levels over the next few days, so I bought a blood glucose monitor — another cost for those keeping track, yay — and turns out that level was just an aberrancy, my blood sugar was fine. But honestly, having to measure several times a day was exhausting, and having to prick a different finger every few hours was not fun. It made me feel for diabetic patients.

Another test I had to do was a head scan to rule out a clot, because that can happen with COVID and it could explain the fog. Luckily, it was negative, but just another test added to the list of things I'd gotten done in the last few months: x-rays, CTs, MRIs, EKGs, echocardiogram, and down the line in April, I had some pulmonary function tests done, as well as an EMG,[16] to test for any neuromuscular abnormalities. All these tests have allowed me to empathize with my patients. I am not claustrophobic, but for some reason, I get a tiny bit anxious when I'm in these machines. Perhaps it was the anticipation of an unknown result that may derail your life. Having to lie down for the tests when I felt like I could barely breathe because of the pleuritis was very uncomfortable. It made all the difference for me when the people performing the tests were friendly and fun.

Finally, there was the cane and the wheelchair. Remember when I was in California and feeling better and thought everything was fine and dandy? That lasted for 11 days, literally the longest stretch of feeling mostly normal that I'd had since meeting 'rona. I still had pleurisy pain, but it was improving.

Well, day 12 came, and I felt tired again, and then day 13 was a little worse. But I thought I was okay enough to go to my appointment alone — highly recommend against that, by the way — and so I started to walk inside Cleveland Clinic main campus. If you've never been there, it's HUGE. I would walk 30 feet and need to sit down and rest. I got around the corner and luckily a good friend that works there saw me and demanded I get a wheelchair.

In addition to shortness of breath and intense knee locking and leg pain, the dizzy spells abruptly set in. While this pain was intense, it wasn't new. The difference is when I'm at home I pretty much stay in bed that day and use a cane to ambulate to the bathroom or if

I need to move for any reason. But when I have places to go, I need a wheelchair. When people saw the wheelchair in the picture I posted, it prompted a very different response. While I completely understand where the outpour of sympathy came from, I really wasn't doing worse than I was before. I point this out not to minimize my symptoms but rather to help others understand why so many people who "seem fine" miss days of work or end up going on disability. What's going on inside someone's body and their physical appearance may very well be completely out of sync.

The Kindness of Caretakers

When I was being wheeled from my appointment back to the parking garage, I had a phenomenal experience. My chauffeur made it a point to stop by every interesting part of the Cleveland Clinic and talk to me about its history. This was such a kind gesture that went a very long way. When you are being wheeled around, you feel a very special kind of vulnerability, and not the good kind of special. If you are in a wheelchair, it means for one reason or another your ability to ambulate is compromised, so not only are you at the mercy of someone else to move you around, but you are also diminutive in stature compared to everyone else. If anyone or anything accidentally falls on you or steps on you, there is not much that you can do about it. It's not a happy feeling. Plus, the chair seats are not padded, so it's just very uncomfortable. For the chauffeur to do all that he did felt like an act of care and love that was very much appreciated. A few days later, I was traveling to Florida to visit my other grandmother and cousin — I mean, when you make it to the east coast, what's one more trip? The person who wheeled me to my gate was also exceptionally kind. Because I had to stand up to go through the security machine, I needed my cane and she made sure another TSA-prescreened cane was brought to me before I stood up. When I was coming back, the person wheeling me was completely detached and I ended up having to stand and lean on the security belt table without a cane or any kind of support for a good three minutes which left my legs screaming at me with pain.

If you are a caretaker in any capacity, remember the power you have over the person you are assisting and remember how vulnerable they are physically. Every decision you make while in their care will affect them.

Finally, I would be remiss if I didn't mention the Walgreens employee who went above and beyond in helping me. The day that I thought I was fine and ended up in a wheelchair, I had driven myself to the Clinic. My dizzy spells presented like vertigo, i.e., they were triggered by head and body movements, so I figured it would be safe for me to drive myself back home as long as I mostly kept my head straight.

Luckily, I was okay to do that, and I had discussed with my mom that if anything changed, I would park on the side of the road, and she would come get me. But before I got home, I knew I was not going to be able to walk and I do not own a wheelchair. I had left my cane in California because when I traveled to Cleveland, I was doing so much better, and mistakenly thought the bad days were behind me.

I stopped by Walgreens and ordered a cane on their app, which they bring to your car. A few minutes later, I got a call from their employee informing me that the cane listed in the app was out of stock, so I ordered a second one and the same thing happened. I explained my situation to her and profusely apologized for my ask, but this woman was an angel. She brought the entire selection of canes to my car and allowed me to choose one and then scan it through the app so I could purchase it because I explained to her that I was too dizzy to walk into the store.

I don't know that woman's name and I honestly don't even remember what she looks like, but she was there for me, and I hope, dear reader, if you or a loved one goes through something, you will have other people there for you, too.

When I recover and am back at work, I will do my best to carry these stories with me every time someone asks for something that seems a bit over the top. Perhaps they have a serious reason that is the root of their request.

Orlando, Florida

We booked our tickets to Florida during my 11-day unicorn stretch and also bought tickets to Universal Studios, because I felt like I deserved a vacation after all this. I really needed the adrenaline rush, and March 2022 was a time when new COVID cases were low in the USA so I figured this was the time. I'd also seen a lot of my friends go to Disney and other such attractions and none of them posted about getting COVID when they got back, so I felt safe in this decision.

When I traveled to Orlando of course, I was in a wheelchair and not doing well. The dizzy spells were at an all-time high, but I tried a new medication, and it actually did wonders for them. After a lot of consideration, and knowing that the tickets my parents paid for were non-refundable, I decided I would go. This was of course after asking my cousin — my park buddy — if he would be okay to push me around all day and he said yes. I knew that some rides may be way too intense for me, but I decided I could just wait those out while he went on them. After all, everything is a give and take, and he was generous enough to push me around all day.

Getting to visit Universal Studios was all worth it. My amazing cousin, Osama, didn't make me feel like a burden at any point. The weather was on our side that day and lots of adrenaline was pumped. That day, for the first time since getting COVID in August, I decided not to wear a mask in public. I truly thought I would be okay with the lower cases and being vaccinated and boosted. I didn't realize that it had been exactly five months on the dot since I had gotten my booster[3] — something notable since Omicron mutates so quickly — but I think that either way I would have not worn the mask since cases were so low.

Unfortunately, your girl got 'rona again

Here's how I think it happened. A lot of the rides had over-the-shoulder restraints that are not sanitized between rides and could have easily had respiratory droplets on them. When my cousin and I went to eat, he used the restroom and therefore washed his hands right before we sat down to eat. I didn't really need to use the restroom and with the burden of being in a wheelchair and having to ambulate with a cane in my fatigued body, I decided I didn't need to go, so I never washed my hands before I ate.

In addition, Florida is very much a no-mask state, at least at the time that I was visiting. The signs at the Orlando airport said to keep three feet apart instead of the recommended six feet. None of the restaurant workers had masks on, so who knows, someone could have been carrying something and that's how I got the virus. There is no way for me to be 100% certain that I got it at Universal or how it happened, but this is just my guess. So, to summarize, I've been keeping away from everyone and everything to the demise of my mental health at certain points, and the day that I take my mask off, I get COVID again… Seems like I've got some lucky stars, don't I?

COVID 2.0

I got back to Ohio on Tuesday night and my leg pain was BAD. I also had terrible indigestion which was weird since I hadn't really had that in a LONG time, perhaps since my initial 40-day stretch with COVID. I did not make the connection. The next day, I woke up feeling like I had daggers in my throat. The congestion, cough, throat soreness, and body aches felt like COVID. The chills I had experienced overnight were a lot more than my regular long-COVID chills that I'd gotten used to living with. My eyes were stinging, something I'd only felt after the COVID vaccine and when I had COVID. I was not thrilled with what I knew that meant.

I took an antigen test and lo and behold it was positive. I messaged my provider, and he told me that even though I'd had several negative repeat tests after my initial infection, I should still do a PCR test to confirm. Well folks, if it looks like COVID, swims like COVID, and quacks like COVID, then it probably is in fact, wait for it … COVID! I was more annoyed than anything else. Does my immune system not work? No one else I was with tested positive, so are some people just more prone to COVID than others? I was happy that no one else got it. I was also bitter, because why me, again? Does this mean I will forever have to wear a mask when everyone else is safe enough to remove it? Yeah, it didn't cripple me this time, but if you work in healthcare, you know for a fact you can't just casually quarantine for 5–10 days every few months or your manager will have some words to say about it. Does this mean my long-COVID will double? No one really knows the answer to any of the above questions. But I decided that it is what it is, and I have to be grateful that I at least qualified for and received one of the novel antivirals. And thankfully for me, it worked, and it worked fast. Maybe the two COVIDs will cancel each other out? Okay, maybe not, but a girl can dream.

A few days later, two out of three family members that I was staying with tested positive. Even though I was isolating, we shared a bathroom. I would wear gloves before touching handles, and then Lysol the crap out of everything I touched, but as we all know by now, it is very hard to not get infected once the virus has made it in the house. I was upset for the two individuals, but I would be lying if I said I wasn't a little relieved. It made me feel like I wasn't a total freak that seemed to get COVID when everyone else was fine. It also meant less restrictions, which was kind of a relief. I didn't have to brush my teeth in my room anymore out of fear of transmitting the virus to others. There is really not much more to say about the second infection. I'm writing this on day nine of 10. I am still having some symptoms, but they are very mild compared to my initial delta infection. The pleurisy is still with me from February and that is challenging, but today it felt like a breakthrough happened. I woke up lying down (I fell asleep sitting) and I noticed that I had no pleurisy pain whatsoever. This is the first time that's happened since I got pleuritis. I don't know if it will last, but I have learned to take the good, no matter how long or short-lived it is.

Life Deferred

Remember when I said I am very passionate about infectious diseases? This passion is not new. In fact, my long-term career goal is to enter an infectious diseases pharmacist role. Long-COVID has put a pin in that. I trust what my providers have been telling me — that I will eventually kick it all because I am improving, albeit very slowly. But because this is all so new, no one can say with certainty if there will be intermittent relapses, or if it'll all be smooth sailing once my symptoms go away. Since I've gotten COVID, many things have been deferred. In addition to not having celebrated my 31st birthday, I missed the camping trip, which was going to be my first-ever. I missed a ski-trip I was hoping to join in Ohio. I missed a baby shower for one of my closest friends. I have had to reschedule my board certification exam twice — the first time was because I was in COVID and this second time is because of the COVID fog that will not be conducive to studying; trust me, I've tried.

I have had to make the decision to remain in community pharmacy instead of continuing to apply for hospital jobs. While I am very proud of my role in the community and I know that any role involving medications will bring me joy, it's not what I specialized in. But I recognize that it is in my best interest to stay close to my parents at a time when my health is so uncertain. I have relied so heavily on them and truly could not have gotten this far without their physical proximity to me. I'm still hesitant when it comes to dating and who to date.

At the end of the day, I have come to realize that my health is the most important part of my life. If I regain full functionality and none of the deferred dreams come true, I am okay with that. I now understand why some terminal patients choose very expensive treatments that only promise six more months of life. Those six months could be the ones that allow them to see a grandchild walk across the stage and accept his diploma, or walk their daughter down the aisle to marry the love of her life, or anything else that is valuable to them. The beauty of long-COVID is that it puts you in so many different circumstances and it's full of uncertainty. You experience a little bit here and a little bit there of many situations that other people go through, and it makes you kinder.

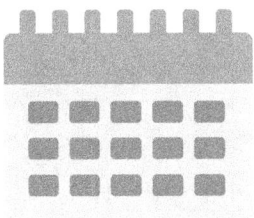

Chapter 7 : April 2022

I finished the first draft of this memoir on March 23, 2022, with a few paragraphs stating my hope for a healthier future, with no real foreseeable end in sight to my long-COVID. I had no idea whether I was ever going to get better. I was picturing a wheel-chair bound life and getting mentally acclimated to that.

I am now writing this at the end of June, and I am so grateful that this fairy-tale of sorts is getting a happy ending after all.

April was filled with even more ups and downs. I started physical therapy (PT) and having to fill out the initial strength-assessment questionnaire was humbling to say the least. Despite having been sick for months, putting on paper that I cannot in fact lift a bag of groceries off the floor was disheartening. I felt more crestfallen than I had when I was in a wheelchair. I was forced to acknowledge my limitations on a medical survey in a way that felt so much more emotionally debilitating than my state disability documents. I know this makes no logical sense, but the act of going through many questions each listing out my myriad of limitations stirred a lot of painful emotions inside of me.

Nevertheless, I was excited. Physical therapy was a step in the right direction. At this stage in my long-COVID, not only were my muscles de-conditioned, I was also losing some of my proprioception, or sense of balance. I began to notice it when I would put my cane on the ground and stumble a little bit. At first, I thought the rubber on the cane itself was getting worn out, but when I would stand and not be able to pinpoint where my feet were positioned relative to my body, or when I'd be walking and my knees would all of a sudden give out under me and I'd nearly fall, I knew it was my balance. I wasn't sure how much physical therapy would help me, but I knew that I had to try everything I could to regain my health.

My physical therapist Tim was so kind and friendly. I was terrified that my concerns wouldn't be taken seriously because it seemed like the whole world was trying to move on from COVID and pretend it no longer existed so we could just put the pandemic behind us. Luckily, I did not experience any of that and it seemed like he was actually very intrigued by my condition as I was his first "official" long-COVID patient. He'd had a few patients that were referred due to muscle weakness that happened after COVID, but I was the first official one. After reviewing my medical history, he wanted to test my strength which is a standard procedure, and boy was I happy I warend him about my mental fog before we started, as it had significantly worsened after COVID 2.0 in March. He told me to outstretch my left arm and I heard that but instead I outstretched my right arm. He paused and then asked for my "other left."

Looking back, it is kind of funny, and I did laugh at the time because I use comedy to defuse tense situations. Internally; however, when I was going through it, I was terrified. Feeling like my brain was always hazy to the extent of not differentiating left from right could be detrimental to my career as a pharmacist. People's lives literally depend on my ability to make critical judgements on the spot. My emotional struggle was exacerbated by my physical limitations. When the physical therapist asked me to do a simple standing knee lift, I was able to get my foot maybe an inch off the ground then had to put it down because of how painful the task was. I literally could not lift my foot. At the end of the session; however, my physical therapist told me that based on his assessment it seemed like the bulk of my weakness was due to inactivity of the muscles as opposed to actual damage which was such a relief to hear, because that meant there was hope for recovery. He also told me that this would be a long road because at that point I'd been fairly inactive for seven months, so naturally, this wasn't something we could rectify in a few sessions. More than anything I appreciated his honesty and I left feeling motivated that it could get better.

Because I knew that I was heading back to Cleveland in a few weeks, I reached out to Dr. Sullivan and asked for a PT referral to the Clinic as well, so I wouldn't miss out on any sessions while I was traveling. I was able to do this swiftly and I am so grateful that I did as you will soon learn why. I do want to first point out my gratitude to Dr. Sullivan for being so patient and providing me with the care that I, like every other patient, deserve. Before getting scheduled in California I had to reach out to him several times because my area is so underserved and the few offices that we have are very oversaturated so I had to keep searching to find a PT office that could accommodate me within a reasonable time frame. I'm so lucky that I found Mad River Sports Medicine and Rehab, but to get there took quite a bit of steps and I'm glad my provider was so responsive.

Reflecting on this makes me a bit sad because I am probably one of the most motivated patients out there. I'm young and have my whole life ahead of me, my condition is projected to improve, I want to go back to work for a myriad of reasons, and I am a healthcare provider who is the child of two healthcare providers — so I come from a very strong background enabling me to successfully navigate the system. Despite all of this, I was getting to my breaking point. Having to reach out to different facilities until I found one that accepted me and my insurance took effort, something I had little of. Having to keep communicating back and forth with my provider was especially stressful because I know how burned out and overworked healthcare providers are, so

I didn't want to be a burden. It took so much mental energy to remind myself that this is my right and I am paying for these services, so yes, it is okay to reach out to my provider several times a week if that is needed for my health. In addition to all of this, discussing costs even with insurance is simply painful. Being on disability means I've been getting half of my normal income and the majority of that goes to pay my medical bills. Going through these experiences makes it so much easier to understand why many patients simply give up on taking care of their health. It's stressful, it's exhausting, at times it feels impossible, and it is SO EXPENSIVE. Certain aspects of my care that were supposed to be covered were denied later on, and my provider was in the process of resubmitting claims and potentially doing a peer-to-peer evaluation with the insurance provider to get those costs covered. I've had to hit pause on paying back my private student loans despite the accruing interest. As a pharmacist, half of my income is still more than a lot of people's full income, but those medical costs may not be a penny cheaper. I don't have a solution to this. The American healthcare system is so complex and broken. I do have an increased understanding of patient behaviors towards healthcare and I will carry that with me when I go back to work.

The Final Trip to Cleveland

My appointments with pulmonology and neurology in March were pushed back to April because I got COVID again. I also had a highly anticipated cardiology appointment that I could not wait to get to. In March, I was diagnosed with something called a patent foramen ovale (PFO),[17-19] i.e., a hole between the top two chambers of the heart. Everyone is born with this hole and in three out of four infants it closes shortly after birth. In the other one out of four individuals, this hole remains present and many go on to live a full and whole-some life blissfully unaware of its presence due to lack of symptoms and complications.

In some people however, it can cause complications like having a stroke. To further complicate things, I found out I have something called factor V leiden (FVL)[20,21] which is a chromosomal mutation in one of the blood's clotting factors, i.e. I have a slightly higher chance of developing a clot in my legs and potentially my lungs. Without going into too much medical jargon, when a person develops a leg clot if it migrates, it moves to the lungs due to the nature of our vasculature. In patients who have a PFO; however, the clot can travel through the top two chambers of the heart, bypassing the lungs and going straight to the brain causing a stroke.

To complicate things even more, after I got COVID in March I was having frequent transient ischemic attacks (TIAs),[22] more commonly known as ministrokes, where my entire left side would go numb for up to 12 hours at a time. The numbness included my face, neck, arm, and leg and it was scary. It is estimated that one out of three people who have a TIA will eventually go on to have a stroke. COVID is associated with strokes. COVID is also associated with increased clotting in general,[23] and knowing that I have FVL means I may be at an even higher risk of a clot which could inevitably migrate to my brain causing a stroke courtesy of my PFO.

At first, I was trying to be okay with all of this information and trust that it would all work out. During one night in particular though, I broke down at the dinner table and told my mom I felt like I was living on borrowed time. That was the night that I found out I have FVL and I was having a rather intense TIA.

My cardiologist at the clinic was pretty amazing. She gave me advice on how to manage my postural orthostatic tachycardia syndrome (POTS) i.e., an abnormal increase in heart rate that occurs after sitting up or standing, secondary to long-COVID, which is why I was initially referred to her. That's what was causing the extreme and sudden changes in my blood pressure and heart rate. She then went on to discuss my PFO, treatment options, and next steps. In the meantime, I would need to get a cardiac MRI, something I was not mentally prepared for.

Medical Exams
The Electromyography Test

In the span of one week, I had three medical tests that proved to be rather laborious for my body. First came the electromyography (EMG) test to assess my nerve and muscle function and to evaluate whether or not there had been any demyelination[24] — damage to the protective covering (myelin sheath) that surrounds nerve fibers — going on. The first 45 minutes consisted of shocks of varying magnitude being delivered to various points of my left leg. Because the goal is to evaluate nerve response, no numbing agent, sedatives, or pain relievers of any kind can be used at the time of the exam. It was excruciating. The last part of the test was called the F wave and I made a joke to the technicians asking if it was called that because of how bad I was about to get effed. I wasn't wrong. That portion consisted of them increasing the magnitude of the shocks until they got a maximal response, after which they shocked me at that level 10 times in a row. I was literally holding on to the strategically placed railing on the wall and wondering if I was better off living with an undiagnosed condition.

After that part was done, I figured the second 45 minutes of inserting needles into my muscles wouldn't be so bad. Oh, was I wrong. Turns out needles being jabbed deeply into your muscles — no matter how small they are — are very painful … and surprise, you bleed. However, the cool part about this exam was I got to hear what my nerve-muscle communication sounds like. At first it sounded like heavy raindrops then it sounded like assault rifles were being fired. There were a few more interesting sounds emanating from the computer monitor that I don't know how to describe very well, but it was definitely a unique experience to actually get to hear that. After the exam was over the attending physician gave an anecdote comparing the pain of the EMG to torture at Guantanamo Bay, so that should really give you a clear idea of how painful it was. Luckily after all that torture, my nerve function was found to be completely intact, so that stormy cloud had a silver lining after all.

The Spirometry Exam

Next came the lung function test. I've never had one done before but I figured how hard could it be to breathe into a tube, especially since my pleuritis was much improved from where it was in February and early March. Well, it turns out when your lungs are tired in any capacity a little bit of exertion can really set you back. Don't get me wrong, if I had tried to complete that test the night I went to the emergency room in February, I probably would have passed out. But it was still very difficult to exert my lungs so forcefully.

I walked out of the exam room, made it to the next lobby, and was waiting to be called in to see the pulmonologist. A minute later the receptionist told me my face was getting abnormally red and asked if I needed water to which I said yes. When I tried to stand, I almost collapsed and they had to get me a wheelchair. It was brutal. My lung function tests came back normal which meant COVID left no permanent structural damage to my lungs. This was great news. It also just meant that the pleuritis was really causing all of my lung symptoms and the pulmonologist said it just takes time and no one knows how long that time will be.

Having to be wheeled out of the pulmonology clinic when I arrived on foot was disheartening. It felt like such a huge step backwards. At this stage of my long-COVID, I had always been carrying my cane just in case I needed it but with a few weeks of physical therapy under my belt, my dizzy spells getting better, and a decline in my POTS episodes — mainly the precipitous drops in blood pressure — I thought I was set on the ambulation front. I felt emotionally numb. I was sad but just didn't have the energy to truly be upset or feel rage or discontent. When you are sick for this long and are being told you will improve, you get to a point of boredom with your condition. I recognize that even having a chance of recovery is a privilege that many with chronic illnesses don't have. That is something I was and will continue to be grateful for. When you are deep in the trenches, though, it's very hard to see the light at the end of the tunnel. You work on accepting your disability for what it is and on not getting your hopes up when you improve because you don't know when the next downtick in health will happen.

The Cardiac MRI

The EMG and spirometry tests really set me back and when that happened, a lot of my symptoms that had been at bay were triggered. I needed a cane to walk around the house, the chills intensified, my pleuritis regressed, and I just felt a generalized weakness that had previously been improving.

I didn't need a wheelchair on the day of my cardiac MRI, but I was so grateful to have my mom with me. My body was very weak, so I rested on a chair and she held my spot in line. It made me feel so much empathy and pain for the patients who don't have someone to accompany them to their appointments. That's the thing about being a patient when you are an empath and a pharmacist. Sometimes the emotional pain is doubled. You feel sad about your circumstances and in being grateful for what you do have, you feel even more sad for those who are less fortunate.

The cardiac MRI had to be one of the worst experiences I've ever had in my life. It's basically a coffin of a machine. Pre-COVID, I never had any issues with small spaces or claustrophobia to any extent. After I got COVID in March; however, I developed some new sensory issues and apparently claustrophobia was one of them. Sitting in a car, for example, became a challenge. Because all of these events were on a relatively abridged time frame, I didn't think to ask for some type of anxiolytic agent and the aftermath was gruesome. I had to lie there for approximately 40 minutes with very loud sounds emanating from the machine, air being blown in my face, heat on my chest (specific to the cardiac component of the test), and literally being trapped in the apparatus. I had to tilt my head to the side the whole time so I could see through the opening behind me in order to mitigate the claustrophobia and it was still very challenging. If I closed my eyes I would picture myself in a coffin falling down into the earth, so not exactly helpful. When I was done, I told my mom that I was done being poked and prodded. I could not handle any more physical tests.

Speech Therapy

Continuing my physical therapy while I was in Cleveland led to the most serendipitous blessing in my long-COVID treatment. My physical therapist Kaitlin went through her entire long-COVID questionnaire with me and asked me if anyone had recommended speech therapy. I didn't even know that was a thing outside of stroke patients or those with speech impediments. She instantly messaged Dr. Sullivan who put in the referral right away and I was able to start my speech therapy journey that afternoon. It was a true game changer.

Now if you are confused about my need for speech therapy, don't worry, I was right there with you. I was referred because of my brain fog which primarily manifested as word-finding difficulty, short-term memory issues, and an overall decline in my acuity. My speech therapist, Abigail, introduced me to how she was going to help me with all that in addition to some of my sensory issues. I was beyond grateful. I was also a little upset as to why no one had suggested this earlier in my course of therapy. My mom reminded me that when I was initially examined, I was doing much better and it seemed like everything was on the up and up, so that is most likely why.

Abigail explained to me how COVID can also present as inflammation in the brain and that was responsible for the fog. She was so gentle with my neurological sensitivities. At one point we had to close the blinds and turn off the lights because getting through a few sentences was enough to give me a pounding headache. This is something I was typically experiencing when trying to do anything involving complex cognitive skills, but lately any sort of thinking or talking would give me a headache. When we did the cognitive assessment test I was thankfully still in the normal range, but it was clear that I didn't have my regular acuity, something I would need to be able to work as a pharmacist. In the few sessions I had with Abigail, she gave me a handful of exercises to help my brain retain words. She also gave me exercises to assist with the sensory overload I had been experiencing. To give you an understanding of what that looks like, sometimes regular conversation was too much. Hearing my own voice was too much. Hearing music in the background or an alarm go off was so overpowering. At best it made it very hard to focus, at worst — which was more often than not — it made me want to rip my face off. These colorful metaphors might sound a bit exaggerated, but they aren't. There is a whole community of long-haulers out there who has the same sensory issues, if not worse than mine.

I'd like to share an exercise that Abigail taught me to get my brain reaccustomed to background nuisances, as working in most pharmacy settings typically entails the phone ringing off the hook. She told me to take an allotted amount of time every day, for example a 20-minute period the first day, and to set repeating alarms in the background. For example, I could be reading or doing the dishes in that 20-minute time frame and have a repeat alarm set to go off every five minutes. This exposure would slowly allow my brain to get accustomed to background noises without feeling so overwhelmed that I need to leave the room or feel like I want to smash the phone. She told me to adjust the exercise based on my response — if 20 minutes with an alarm every five minutes proves to be too much, the next day I could do a 15-minute interval with an alarm every seven minutes, for example. As my tolerance improves, I would learn to gradually shorten the interval of the alarms, for example every two minutes in a 20-minute time stretch. As challenging as this exercise was at first, it proved to be incredibly helpful. I later discovered that there are earbuds that are sold specifically to attenuate noise without eliminating it, so fellow long-haulers I encourage you to look into that option as well.

Tough Decisions

After completing all of my initially scheduled appointments at the Cleveland Clinic I was faced with some tough decisions to make. Getting a PFO closure procedure scheduled isn't so cut and dried. It required a few more appointments and this all meant time in Cleveland, i.e., more money spent on renting a car. While my parents were graciously paying for this, I felt bad wasting any money. In addition, after the procedure I would need to have follow-up visits after one month, six months, and one year which would not be feasible assuming I would be back at work in the West Coast. I also missed my life in California. My books, my apartment, my cat, all of it. Being in Cleveland was pivotal for my health, but I was literally just passing time between appointments. I also recognized that my mom's life was literally put on hold to accompany me to all my appointments over the last few months. Without her there is literally no way I could have done any of it, and I didn't want to keep burdening her any more than I needed to, despite her insistence that I wasn't.

I knew that I had the option to continue my PFO care at Stanford. The determining factor would be whether or not I would have access to speech therapy. My provider, Patricia, immediately put in the referral and when I called to schedule my appointment the scheduler said she had to run it by the therapist first. Given how remote we are, there was only one speech therapist at the time, so she was only accepting critical patients. I am happy to report that she accepted me as a patient given that my job is completely cerebral, and I made the decision to go back to California.

Self-Acceptance

As fate would have it, one of my best friends was getting married in Cleveland at the end of April and I was happy to be able to attend her wedding. By this time, I was starting to recover from all the medical exams and the day started off okay. By noon; however, I was having intense chills and dizzy spells and my body was so weak. I was faced with a really tough decision to make. On the one hand she is one of my best friends who drove four hours during her medical residency to attend my pharmacy school graduation. On the other hand, my health was suffering. I was physically exhausted. This was also going to be my first large group outing since I had become disabled, and I didn't know how others would react to seeing me in a cane. I take pride in being fashionable and stylish and just looking after my appearance in general. Using a cane could change that.

I decided that this friendship meant more to me than how others would perceive me and I knew that I would be sitting the majority of the time so I would make it work. I had a second cup of coffee that day — something I haven't done in months — and put on a little bit of makeup and headed towards the wedding venue. Of course, I showed up a little late which is something that would never happen historically, but by this stage I had learned to give myself grace and accept my limitations.

I was one of very few people wearing a mask at the wedding. I felt a little insecure. Everyone there was vaccinated and health conscious. Still, I had an active PFO and I could not take any level of risk, so even in my picture with the bride, I kept the mask on. Luckily, everyone there was so incredibly friendly. So much that people kept offering to bring me drinks and desserts to the table. If this had happened a few months ago, I would have been mortified and refused. But now I know how to accept the help, so I gladly accepted their kind gestures. When I wasn't able to finish my slice of cake because my chills started to intensify preventing me from effectively holding my fork, I put it down and accepted my new reality gracefully. I was grateful for the half slice that I was able to enjoy.

Although I didn't want to harsh everyone's mellow and talk about long-COVID, it was near impossible for it not to come up. People ask about your job, if you are visiting Cleveland, etc., and so I had to mention it. This was a very enlightening moment for me. Up until this point, I was a little surprised with how so many people had disregarded mask wearing all together. Now, I'm not here to tell you what to do, I'm simply stating how I was feeling. Even as I write this in June in the "post-pandemic" timeframe, the USA is averaging 100,000 new cases daily, so COVID is certainly not gone. My physical and speech therapists in

Cleveland told me they see many patients, young and old, in my position, so it seemed curious that people wouldn't be afraid of getting long-COVID. Even one of my providers stated that she was more scared of getting long-COVID than COVID itself.

In talking to people at the wedding, I found out that many people have never even heard of long-COVID. In a way that put things into perspective for me. If I thought that getting COVID meant at worst five days of feeling a little congested, for example, I would certainly abandon any mask-wearing practices I had because it wouldn't be worth the hassle. Overall, I was grateful that I was able to share my experience and learn about other points of view. Sadly, things with COVID have been highly politicized and it's easy to get caught up in the weeds of it all. When we keep an open mind and give everyone a voice, it makes understanding each other a little bit easier.

I had a blast at the wedding, but I wasn't able to dance and that was really gut wrenching. You're probably rolling your eyes thinking that dancing should be the least of my concerns after all that I've been through, but it isn't. I'm Middle Eastern and dancing is in our blood. I've been a dancer since I was 13 years old. I even had a Zumba teaching certificate. It's how I have a good time. Sitting at the table while bobbing my head to the music and watching everyone else on the dance floor was bittersweet. It was the first time I'd felt attractive in months and being in the presence of others was FUN! It was also a little challenging because as I sat there, I didn't know if I would ever truly be able to dance again. I decided to enjoy what I could and make peace with the painful emotions because all of it is part of my journey.

After the wedding, my friend told me that she really wanted me to be a bridesmaid but knew how challenging that would be with long-COVID. My friend absolutely made the right decision because as I described up until an hour before the wedding, I wasn't sure I was going to make it, and I showed up late. I bring this up because it is a perfect anecdote to illustrate what people mean when they say they are grieving their chronic illnesses. It isn't always about the physical pain caused by the illness itself. It also encompasses the missed opportunities and special moments that are a side effect of the chronic illness.

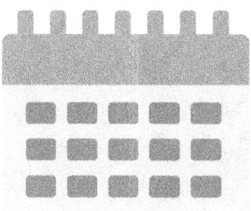

Chapter 8 : May 2022

When I went back to California one of my flights was approximately five hours long. I had been mildly limping that morning, but I was able to ambulate without a cane. The more time I spent on the plane the weaker my legs started to feel. Soon my muscles were aching and when the plane ride was over, I couldn't take a step without the cane. So, when I walked into physical therapy with the cane a few days later, my therapist was just as surprised as I was. Surprised because when I left for Cleveland I had been doing better.

I was in a bit of an emotional state that day, not only because I was needing a cane again, but also because I didn't know what these ups and downs would mean for my career. Do I just give up and find a remote job? That's not what I want to do, I love the clinical component of my work–many clinical roles are not remote–and I love talking to people. But if my health wasn't going to support that, at what point do I call it and accept this as my permanent reality?

Luckily for me, Tim was very insightful. He told me that he suspected that the long plane ride along with all those back-to-back strenuous exams set my body back a little bit, but that we would be able to tell within a few sessions whether that was a circumstantial lapse, or if it's something that will continue to ebb and flow. He also told me that when considering my job options, it's best to look at the fluctuation intervals in my health moving forward. For example, evaluating how long it takes me to recover from this nadir compared to how long it used to take, and seeing when the next relapse happens. This advice was so helpful because I was really conflicted about what to do with my life. Disability is inconvenient at any stage in life, but when you are at the beginning of your career and have hundreds of thousands of dollars in student loans to pay off, it makes things especially sticky. After receiving his advice, I decided to breathe, focus on my session, and take it one day at a time. My disability had been extended to the middle of August, so I knew I still had some time to figure things out.

In the meantime, I was getting ready for speech therapy in Eureka, CA with Kayla and I was very nervous before our first session. Despite never having been personally gaslit in the medical arena I was still nervous because this was a very niche treatment for my long-COVID fog that I didn't even know existed until very recently. Furthermore, I was already improving from when I had started speech therapy in Cleveland and on that particular day of my appointment my brain felt very clear. Much like the many other symptoms I've had, it's always an up and down, i.e., some days are terrible and some days are really good. What if Kayla thought I was exaggerating my condition and decided to discharge me? I knew that I couldn't just keep going back and forth to Cleveland indefinitely for treatment. I decided that the only way to find out was to go to the appointment and see for myself. A few sentences into our conversation about my condition were enough to reassure me that Kayla was on my side, and we were going to work together to get my brain in the best condition possible.

What I appreciated about Kayla is that she listened to me and trusted the information I was giving her. For example, describing how my fog worsens as the day progresses prompted her to make all my future appointments in the afternoon so she could see me at my worst in order to provide me with maximal benefit. We worked on retraining my brain to get used to routine and structure in order to get back to work. We worked on going to the grocery store. I may have done this once after getting COVID very early on and that was it. Going to the grocery store was a terrifying experience for me because I don't know when I'll get a dizzy spell or when my blood pressure is suddenly going to drop. What if it happened as I was reaching for celery on a shelf in the produce section and I fell over? How would I ambulate with my cane and a cart? And these are all fears for when I'm not in a wheelchair. These were all valid and legitimate concerns that persisted even when I was starting to improve. So, Kayla helped me get past them and make that big move of going to the grocery store. I felt victorious. Over the next few weeks my health improved at a staggeringly high rate. I found myself remembering random pharmacology concepts and being able to articulate them without any trepidation. I ditched the cane and my dizzy spells and POTS episodes were negligible. It truly felt like I was turning over a new leaf. Tim got me set up with different machines that I would be able to use at the gym once I graduated PT and Kayla told me that I could keep coming to speech therapy until I felt ready. In the meantime, I had met with Dr. Sharma, the interventional cardiologist at Stanford, and we decided to move forward with my PFO closure procedure.

As you've probably picked up on by now, I like to be prepared for worst-case scenarios. This was heightened by things occurring to me that are not as common like being diagnosed with FVL. Being prepared gives me some sense of control over my life, so while I did not have any reason to suspect a metal allergy I wanted to find out before the PFO occluder device was permanently inserted in my heart. There is a great website called www.sensiband.com and they sell home allergy tests so patients can ensure they are good to go before any hip/knee replacement surgeries, or any surgeries warranting placement of a foreign metal. Now you may need to be evaluated by a specialist to be cleared prior to a procedure if there is reason to suspect an allergy, but if you are just hyper-cautious like me, the bands are a simpler way to find out if you have allergies. Fortunately, I found out that I am not allergic to any of the three metals in the occluder device so I just had to get to June 1, 2022, aka the day of my procedure, and some semblance of normalcy would finally be restored to my life. In the few weeks leading up to the procedure, things really changed all around me. It seemed like as a nation we were so eager to move past COVID that many people were simply acting like it no longer existed despite our continued average of ~100,000 new daily cases. I understood the urge; however, as someone who was having regular TIAs I had to protect myself from getting a new COVID infection at all costs, because a new COVID infection could mean a stroke and permanent debilitation. I stopped eating out or even getting Starbucks because many restaurant employees no longer wore masks and I didn't want to be the victim of an asymptomatic carrier. I even wore a mask in front of my family members if I knew they were hanging out with other people. While this is a challenging and restrictive way to live, it's important to showcase why many people still mask when the majority have stopped. People have underlying conditions that are not physically apparent. Other people live with immunocompromised patients. Some people got long-COVID and it's only gotten worse, or it got better but they don't want to live through it again.

It's important that this is kept in mind because everyone has the right to protect themselves. I had someone tell me that she got a rock thrown at her for wearing a mask in a restaurant. Meanwhile, in other places, many people still mask, especially indoors, because people there don't perceive another person's choice to mask as a personal affront to their freedom. That goes to show how politicized the pandemic has become, which is truly outrageous.

My takeaway from all of this is that it's important not to verbally confront people — and it goes without saying not to physically assault them — for wearing a mask because not wanting to get COVID is reason enough, especially if they have other medical conditions. It's also important to recognize that humans can only endure so much restriction and many people don't have the capacity to stay masked up forever because that's not how we were made. So, while I'm always surprised when I see a cancer patient on chemotherapy going about their activities without a mask, I recognize that they probably know the risk they are putting themselves at and that is their prerogative. If we could all accept that different people will make different decisions and that is okay, the world would be a much better place.

Happy Endings & New Beginnings

The week leading up to my procedure was filled with joy and anxiety. I graduated from both physical therapy and speech therapy and I felt like I was ready to take on the world again. I was also really nervous about my procedure. I knew that the benefit outweighed the risk, but like many procedures, there is a chance, albeit very small, of death. After extensive discussions with my parents, I decided to tell my other family members about the PFO and the upcoming procedure. While I knew the chance of any complication was negligible, I figured that if the roles were reversed, I would much rather know ahead of time that my relative was undergoing a procedure instead of later finding out that they passed and all of it being a complete and utter shock. So, I told everyone close to me that I loved them, and I got ready for the drive down to Stanford. I would be remiss if I didn't take a moment to mention the generosity of my friends Joann and Taavi. I became friends with them less than two years ago, when I moved to California, and yet the kindness I've seen from them is one of a kind. When I was telling Joann about my PFO and the drive down to Stanford, a six-hour drive with gas prices nearing seven dollars a gallon, she told me that she and her husband, Taavi, had points for a four-day stay at a hotel in Palo Alto-the city of the hospital. At first, I wanted to decline, simply because that was such a generous offer, but when I looked at my financial situation — for reference as I'm writing this at the end of June, I have $139 in my bank account — I decided to accept their generous gift. Those four nights were such a tremendous help, especially after all of the medical expenses I have incurred. Joann and Taavi, you are wonderful people, and from the bottom of my heart, thank you.

If you are disabled because of long-COVID or any other illness and you have friends and family offering help in your life, I recommend you accept it. It took me months to get here, but I wish I had learned to accept the help sooner.

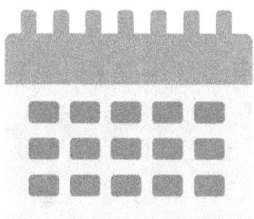

Chapter 9 : June 2022

The Procedure

On June 1, 2022, I woke up at five am, prayed, brushed my teeth, took the aspirin pill I was instructed to take, got dressed, and hyperventilated for an hour or so before it was time to go to my procedure. Because of continued COVID precautions, my mom, who had driven down with me, wasn't allowed to stay in the waiting area so I gave her one final hug goodbye before I went into the pre-op room. I was beyond nervous, but I knew that Dr. Sharma, my operating cardiologist, is the head of interventional cardiology at Stanford, so I was literally in the best possible hands.

When I was taken into the procedure room the team warned me that the lidocaine injection might hurt a little, and my response was nothing would hurt after the EMG test, which proved to be quite true, so there's that silver lining. The procedure involved two different catheters going in through the groin which is classified as minimally invasive, so I only underwent light sedation. It definitely took the edge off, but I was actually wide awake and my follow-up appointment with Dr. Sharma proved that I really did remember everything clearly. When the catheter made its way up to the right atrium, I was able to see it attempting to go through into the left atrium, but to no avail. Dr. Sharma then did several bubble studies — how a PFO is diagnosed — and one with the Valsalva maneuver just to be certain, and yet no bubbles crossed to the other side. So basically, there was no PFO. If you didn't see that one coming trust me... neither did I.

The procedure left me processing a lot of different feelings. Relief that I wouldn't have to be on two antiplatelet medications for a certain amount of time. Relief that I didn't have a device implanted inside of me. Relief that I didn't have a hole in my heart that was increasing my chance of strokes. I was also annoyed because even though there was no PFO, the catheters had punctured the groin, so I still had the same painful recovery for a few days. In the grand scheme of heart procedures, it's not that big of a deal; however, the fact that it was unnecessary was frustrating.

I was also befuddled. Extensive testing and imaging had been done prior to the procedure by cardiologists at the Cleveland Clinic and Stanford, two of the top institutions in cardiac care globally. Had the healthcare providers failed me? Most importantly, PFO or not, I was having TIAs, so does that mean those were all triggered by long-COVID? I felt like I had to take matters into my own hands, so I immediately scheduled a follow-up appointment with Dr. Sharma. I didn't know if the actual echocardiogram and MRI had transferred over from the Clinic or if he'd only had access to the written report, so I kept on calling different departments at the Clinic until I was able to transfer an actual copy of the imaging itself to Stanford. It's not that I didn't trust the judgment of the physician. It's simply that I was told there was a hole, and when we went inside my heart, there was no hole. I needed answers.

Answers to My Skepticism

My follow-up with Dr. Sharma was very enlightening. It provided me with much needed comfort. It turns out that he did have access to the imaging prior to the procedure. We discussed how the results of the MRI weren't very definitive. We discussed how the initial bubble study wasn't a strong positive, meaning it appeared as though there were trace bubbles.

However, that can happen sometimes with the rationale involving late return through the pulmonary circuit or something to that effect — I am not an interventional cardiologist so keeping up with the nitty gritty details was a bit challenging. Given the big picture, undergoing the procedure and finding out there was no PFO was a much safer alternative than saying the results weren't definitive and waiting for a stroke to happen. Dr. Sharma also informed me that the suspect TIAs were likely due to my long-COVID, so I would need to follow up with the long-hauler clinic.

Reflecting back on this experience is very sobering. Though I'm a clinically trained pharmacist and truly have never had a reason not to trust any of my healthcare providers, I was still skeptical for a minute because I didn't have all the answers. It made me understand why so many patients unfortunately lose trust in the healthcare system and decide to completely forfeit their health. Some things in medicine aren't so cut and dried, and for many patients, especially those who have no health training, that is a tough pill to swallow.

Couple that with past experiences of potential gaslighting from some healthcare providers and you have a recipe for full-on mistrust of the system. If someone is already feeling skeptical of the healthcare they are receiving and is required to pay thousands of dollars to pay for an outcome they are not guaranteed, it is easy to understand why that person might decide that it's not worth it. These kinds of experiences can be very traumatizing for some patients. Some people may even wonder if their experiences were due to racial or religious prejudices. This is why it is crucial for providers to take the time and explain nebulous concepts to their patients so that they don't lose faith in the healthcare system from one quizzical or at times truly negative encounter.

Ebb and Flow

I'm a fighter until the very end, and despite the many times I've wanted to give up I haven't and I won't. Having said that, dealing with all of this has been challenging. On top of the obvious physical and emotional challenges, managing and coordinating the numerous appointments has not been an easy feat. Yes, being on disability theoretically gives me all the time in the world, but there's a reason why I'm on disability.

Having an unreliable body that decides to give out at any given moment, or start vomiting in public when I am incapable of rushing to a restroom, or present me with a brain fog so thick that I can't even remember to check my calendar to see if I have any appointments, makes it very challenging to schedule, coordinate, and keep those appointments. There was a time frame when I started forwarding everything to my mom, because I had a few instances where I would read the appointment as 11:30 am, yet somehow it would translate to 1 pm in my brain, for example. Or the time when I had to reschedule my brain CT, because I forgot that I wasn't supposed to eat before the procedure.

As time went on and my fog started to lift, keeping track of those appointments became easier. I'm also very fortunate that I never forgot to pay my bills, but keeping track of all of it was still challenging. If you have long-COVID, one thing that worked for me was having a physical to-do list front and center in the living room (or any space you know you will frequent) and immediately adding all of my appointments to my phone calendar with several reminder alarms.

The alarms would be set far enough in advance so that if I had completely forgotten about the appointment, I would have enough time to get ready and drive to said appointment. Even now writing all of this is a bit painful. It triggers so much vulnerability and memories of a time when I, an adult with a doctorate degree, had a diminished intellectual bandwidth. It makes me proud of and grateful for how far I've come. I also realize that I am truly blessed.

I believe in God and I am so grateful to Him for getting me this far. Whether you believe in a higher power or not, we can all agree that for one reason or another, some people improve and some people do not, and it is challenging to see yourself improve while leaving others behind. One concrete example was a video reel I was conflicted about posting on my long-hauler chronicles Instagram page. On the one hand, I wanted to chart my improvement because the point of the page was to share my journey. On the other hand, I was feeling guilty because so many of the long-COVID friends I have made through that page are in much worse shape than I am, and the last thing I wanted to do was rub my improvement in their faces. I ended up sharing the reel along with those feelings in the caption. I was overwhelmed by the kindness shared by my fellow long-haulers. Many of them shared how seeing any improvement in others actually comforts them because it lets them know that there is hope. If you've made it this far, thank you for letting me share my journey with you. My biggest power is in raising awareness for long–COVID and spreading compassion for long–haulers. I'm at a stage where many people think my PASC is over because of how far I've come along and because I say I'm doing so much better. In reality, I still wake up to chills almost every single day.

They do tend to go away after about 30 minutes which is a tremendous improvement from where I was at. Every few weeks the fog will rear its ugly head not so much in a way that hinders my critical thinking ability, but rather I'll want to say a word and feel like I need to verify its meaning before I commit to it. My left side still goes numb a lot, though now it's mostly just my left arm as opposed to complete numbness from my face through my foot. My pleuritis and insomnia still like to remind me that they are there lurking in the background, though the frequency and magnitude of their presence are negligible compared to where they were in February.

I still have other things here and there that I deal with, but overall, I can at least live like this. I think that having been vaccinated and boosted, the passage of sufficient time, as well as the antiviral I received after my second infection have been key factors in my improvement.

Because I live in California and plan on going back to work very soon, I was officially referred to the long-COVID clinic at Stanford. The first available appointment was either virtual, scheduled one month out, or if I wanted an in-person it was two and a half months out. This is not a slight against Stanford, but rather it's to show how impacted the long-COVID clinics are across the nation because of how many people have been affected in one way or another from COVID. My appointment will be at the beginning of August, and I look forward to receiving more answers on my suspect TIAs as well as lingering symptoms. Once that appointment is over, I plan on returning to work full time and I cannot be more thrilled.

Having this sudden improvement has been a bit scary. When I was fully disabled, I was sad, but I also felt very nurtured and taken care of. Now that I'm very close to my baseline again, that feeling of being sheltered is gone and I feel like I went from being a toddler to an adult overnight. I've been on disability for almost a year and the world didn't stop and wait for me. There's a level of anxiety that accompanies going back to work and essentially re-learning pharmacy. I feel very fortunate that I still have some time on disability and that my fog is gone so I can be prepared for work when I'm back. Not everyone has the same timeline of symptom improvement that I do, so if you have a co-worker that seems a little overwhelmed when they first come back, be gentle, it can be very scary for someone to transition back into the real world.

If you are interested in finding out more about my journey, I will continue to post updates on my Instagram page@longhaulerchronicles. For now, this is the end of my journey. If you, dear reader, are interested in sharing yours, I would love it if you reach out through my Instagram page.

I have heard from so many people across the globe who unfortunately have similar or even worse stories than myself, and it seems like just sharing with each other has been a little cathartic.

My biggest advice to you if you are going through it is that when life gives you mold, make sure to make some penicillin out of it. As hard as it is, and believe me I know, try to see the beauty where you can.

Most importantly, never ever stop advocating for yourself. I've heard so many stories of gaslighting with regards to long-COVID. Keep fighting and keep searching for providers who validate your very real condition. There are many support groups on Facebook with a lot of room for Q&A. There is a vast community of long-haulers on Instagram that you can connect with. Never give up. Never give in.

Hopefully, we will all look back one day and say it certainly passed…

It may have passed like a kidney stone, but it did in fact pass.

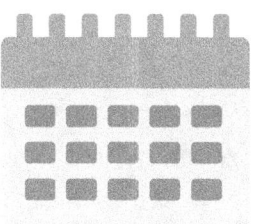

Chapter 10 : Final Thoughts

Other Disabilities

I've talked a lot about empathy, but I really cannot stress how much my heart goes out to those who have it worse. Some people have had much more intense PASC symptoms than myself and for a much longer amount of time. I've learned to recognize why some quadriplegics choose to go for death with dignity. I know people have different beliefs on this, and I am not even presenting my own. I am simply saying, I understand why someone who is unable to do anything without the assistance of others may no longer see a reason to live in the world; why they may choose to do something that others may think is extreme.

I've also learned to empathize with patients who had to be hospitalized with restrictions and no family members allowed to visit them. I had to go through this for 14 days while I was in the comfort of my home. My heart goes out to all those people who lost their loved ones and were not able to see them for one final goodbye.

I've even learned to empathize with people who don't think we should wear masks under any situation. While my story should give reason to believe that masks do work, I can say that since I've gotten pleuritis, wearing a mask has been challenging. Sometimes I feel like I truly cannot breathe with it on, so I get why others are inclined to never want to wear it, regardless of the risk present in any particular situation.

I've learned that being open about my health is what works best for me, but this approach does not work for everyone. Some people need to believe that their condition is not actually as bad as it is to move forward. No one has the right to tell someone how to process their grief or illness. The best thing we can do is to do our best to be there for each other and ask our loved ones how we can support them in any way that they need.

I've learned that many people have health problems and do not want anyone to know, and this is their right. Health is a very private issue, and unfortunately, we live in a stigma-riddled world, so sharing health issues can mean putting a lot of things at risk — including employment status.

If you have people in your life that don't share these things with you, try to not take it personally. I say this while fully acknowledging that this is a daily struggle for me, because I want my friends and family to share things with me so that I can be there for them. However, it's important to constantly remind ourselves that it's not always about us. It's also important to keep this in mind because sometimes we reach out to people and don't hear back. While we won't know if they don't share, they really might be going through something of their own.

Friendships

I would be remiss if I didn't explain a few things regarding friendships. You've read a lot of statements here about my "friends," but I want to clarify that my circle of close friends are amazing people who have been there for me through all of this and continue to be to this day. While there certainly are some people I thought were closer friends than they proved to be, I am very blessed with an inner circle of friends that I would never change for the world. If there is anything I have learned through this year, it is that we all have different needs, and it's not fair to expect people to know what we want just because we are close. I've learned to communicate my needs. Even if it's for something as simple as asking someone to send me a card.

When I'm busy with work and not sick, I often forget to text people back the same day, sometimes even a few days later. I try to keep this perspective in mind when I'm on the flip side to minimize my own pain of taking it personally and feeling like the said friend doesn't care about me. I have also learned how painful it is to be vulnerable and chronically sick, so I try to do better.

A few months ago, I royally messed up. A friend's mom passed away, and because our primary mode of communication is WhatsApp, I only saw the first few words of her second message — I have my phone settings set to not be able to preview texts. This was during the heart of my COVID, and her second text gave no clue to the context of the first one, which talked about her mom's passing.

When I opened the message a few months later, I was mortified. I had let a friend down in a terrible way. I profusely apologized, sent her flowers, and vowed to do better with all my friends. Similarly, a colleague and her family got COVID, and during our text exchange, I got busy with my own symptoms and forgot to text back for a few weeks. Even so, I did eventually text her back and checked in on her.

I know I'm not perfect and I never will be, just like no human is. Sometimes people really do care, but they have their own things going on and forget to respond. Sometimes people really don't care and when their actions prove that, it's important to not keep holding a space for them in our hearts because that will only cause us more pain.

The people who have things going on in their lives and still remember us and make time to reach out, those people are gold and it's important that we communicate our appreciation to them. I am so blessed to have a handful of friends that are like that. I am blessed that when I'm needing more attention and care than usual, I feel comfortable enough to communicate that need to them, despite their own busy lives.

I am grateful to have amazing family members in the states and overseas who somehow seem to prioritize reaching out to me no matter what they are going through. Believe me, if you knew what my family overseas goes through, we would sit together and cry for days, because I at least have never had to go 30 hours without electricity.

I hope that you all have at least one or two people in your lives that make you feel loved. If you don't, I'm sorry. Hopefully, other wonderful people come into your lives soon. This book is my attempt at making everyone who's struggling feel loved.

How to Be a Ray of Sunshine in a Long-Hauler's Life

Below are some tips on how to be there spectacularly for people you know who may be experiencing really bad long-COVID or another disability. I also incorporate some advice for the patients, based on my experiences and things I've learned. Keep in mind that these are all ways that work for me and I'm a highly social extrovert who loves to express things and talk about my feelings. These may not work for everyone, and if you know for a fact that loving someone like this will suffocate them, then please follow what you know and take my advice with a grain of salt.

1. Check on your friends and family regularly, and by that, I mean every day to once every two weeks depending on the relationship, the proximity you have with that person, and their need for space and communication preferences. It helps tremendously to know that others are thinking of you, especially if you aren't the life of the party anymore or able to physically be there with them.

2. Validate their feelings and symptoms. Sometimes they may think they are going crazy because the symptoms are so wild and all over the place. They are not. This reassurance may help.

3. Don't compete with them. It's absolutely okay to share experiences, especially if you got COVID, but if you aren't going through it, please be mindful not to make it about you. You also don't want to make them resentful for not having recovered as quickly as you did, since none of it is within our control.

4. If someone posts about their pain and you don't comment, like, or interact in any way with their post, do not bring it up later in a random conversation that has nothing to do with the patient's illness. Because then you are letting the patient know that you did in fact see that they were sick, but you didn't care enough to say anything, and that's just hurtful.

5. Ask the patient how you can help and bring up examples, like taking out their trash, grocery shopping for them, getting them flowers, cleaning their cat's litter box, taking their dog for a walk, providing financial assistance, or setting up a GoFundMe where possible and if needed. This will show them that you are not providing empty promises and will encourage them to actually ask for the help they need. In a nutshell, treat it like a real grievance because even though they may have not lost anyone, they could be losing their health and therefore need very similar assistance.

6. Casseroles shouldn't only be reserved for families of the dead. This may depend on whether the patient lives alone or with family, but it may genuinely be life-altering for them. If I could go back and do it again, I would take up my neighbor's profuse pleas to take out my trash. I would also take up my friends on their offers of bringing me food and towels. If you are in it now, let people be there for you.

7. Laugh with them. Sometimes some of life's most painful moments should be handled with an air of levity. Just make sure you aren't being insensitive. It's truly a fine line.

8. Grieve with them. Don't minimize their fears. Don't dismiss them. They are going through pain, and ignoring or denying it will not help them.

9. Send them a card. It's kind of embarrassing to ask for this, but trust me, it will mean the world to them. And maybe flowers, or chocolates, or a care package of any sort. Or DoorDash some tea to them.

10. My family in Syria who is living without electricity or water sent me gifts to commemorate this prolonged illness and it meant the WORLD to me. Similarly, some of my family members in the USA did the same. It really made me feel better because no matter what, there is a deep level of pain when you are so sick for this long, and gifts mean they are thinking of you and love you, and that helps.

11. If your friend's physical capacity has been severely restricted, FaceTime them or take pictures of activities you'd normally do together and take time to share those moments with them. For example, if you were planning a hiking trip that they can no longer attend, FaceTime them while there or take pictures and show them when you get back.

12. Do not tell them "It's all about staying positive" because not only is that not true, you are inadvertently laying a guilt trip on them. If they don't get better, it must mean they weren't positive enough. If they are positive and don't get better, were you lying? It's very unrealistic and unhelpful advice. There is more and more evidence showing that in PASC, COVID affects the autonomic nervous system and that's what's causing a lot of the symptoms, so how will a positive outlook help that? I have been very optimistic and experienced painful episodes afterwards, and I've been incredibly pessimistic and had bouts of improvement, so please for the love of all things sacred, do not leave people with that guilt trip and the false promise of a clean bill of health with a "positive attitude."

13. Do not shame them. Maybe they didn't wear a mask that day and they happened to hit the COVID jackpot. But who among us hasn't taken off the mask at all since March of 2020? Not many people, that's for sure. They may have done everything right and gotten it. They may have not. What I can say is, no one thought we would be in it for this long and it gets really dark, so maybe they made a decision based on their mental health that day and ended up with COVID. It sucks, but that doesn't mean they deserve to be shamed. Don't be like the guy scheduling my medical appointment who told me, "You're a healthcare provider, you should have known better" … thanks, Karen.

14. Some of you may be reading this and thinking, "Man, my friend got sick months ago, I forgot to reach out and now I'm just embarrassed." I actually had a very close friend admit this to me. I'm here to tell you to reach out. If you are close, every day that goes by deepens the wedge between you guys. If you aren't close, it may not bother them as much, but it may make them question the relationship. I can guarantee they will only be grateful if you reach out.

Common PASC Symptoms Experienced by Friends

I want to include this section because I realize that my case is extreme. Not everyone with PASC will end up on disability, but many people who get it will experience some symptoms. There are other symptoms that I did not experience, but others certainly have, so below I share a list of symptoms my friends have mentioned :

1. It seems like brain fog is very prevalent, especially presenting as forgetfulness for a lot of people. Write things down, set timers right away, and try to use established routines. For example, if you hang your keys in a certain spot when you get home, make sure to always use that spot. It makes it easier to find them when you lose them. Sometimes I would go into a different room of my house to do something, and by the time I got there, I would have forgotten why I went there. A friend of mine shared a similar experience. Some providers recommend select vitamins, but to my knowledge, at the time that this is being written, there is no full–blown "cure" for brain fog. Speech therapy definitely helped. But if you find that you are forgetting things, can no longer access your visual memory, or are misplacing items, I'm sorry, and you aren't alone. It stinks and it's happening to a lot of people. Hopefully time makes it a little better.

2. Diarrhea or stomach disturbances in general. Mine lasted for maybe three months. Now the upset is not as frequent. I know quite a few people who kept going through this for a month or so after their COVID infections. It stinks — literally — and medications may help, but before you drive yourself crazy wondering what's going on with your diet, it may be long-COVID.

3. Intrusive anxiety. A friend of mine had thoughts like "What if I wake up and find my husband dead next to me?" For me, it was a laundry list of things, but one very personal example occurred when I was talking to a guy. At the time we weren't exclusive, and my thoughts were "What if he happens to match with my other single friend and they end up together and then I get excluded from all the friend groups because it's easier for everyone that way to avoid an awkward dynamic?"

That scenario probably sounds very ludicrous and unlikely, and it is. But here's the thing, they all go back to feeling isolated. My therapist helped me realize that the reason these insecurities surface in parallel to my physical symptoms is because when my health deteriorates, it's deteriorating alone, i.e., no one else around me is having the same issues. So, it's natural for my brain to fear losing my sole caretaker. It's natural to have anxieties rooted in feeling ousted and isolated because that's how I am when I'm losing my health. Other people may be nice, but I'm still disabled and reliant on others. One mantra she gave that helps me is "My thoughts are caused by my anxiety, which is valid because my health is deteriorating alone. But they are just thoughts, and just because I think them does not mean they are or will become my reality."

4. Changes in sexual function. I have had some friends state that they have not been able to achieve an orgasm since they got COVID and their providers told them that it is all related to COVID's effects on the autonomic nervous system, but it will all come back in time.

All these symptoms should hopefully demonstrate how different long-COVID or PASC can present for different people. So, if you got COVID and are having strange symptoms, you could be experiencing long-COVID. Not everyone who gets it will have as many symptoms as I do, but it does affect many people who get COVID with the current estimates in the literature ranging from 5%–80%. These numbers may change in the future, but they are reflective of the current literature and guidance at the time this book is being written.

Notes

We have been living with COVID-19 for over two years now and I trust that the reader will have no problem researching some of the medical things I have stated in this book for accuracy. Referencing every study or body of literature addressing COVID and long-COVID would require a book in and of itself, so I will present a few references that I think are beneficial.

If you are interested in more personal stories of long-COVID, I recommend you search the term "long-COVID" on Amazon, as the number of books in this area continues to grow.

References

1. Coronavirus Disease 2019 (COVID-19). Centers for Disease Control and Prevention. Accessed August 28, 2022. https://www.cdc.gov/coronavirus/2019-ncov/index.html

2. Post-COVID Conditions: Overview for Healthcare Providers. Centers for Disease Control and Prevention. Updated July 9, 2021. Accessed August 28, 2022. https://www.cdc.gov/coronavirus/2019-ncov/hcp/clinical-care/-post-covid-background.html

3. Post-COVID Conditions: Overview for Healthcare Providers. Centers for Disease Control and Prevention. Updated July 9, 2021. Accessed August 28, 2022. https://www.cdc.gov/coronavirus/2019-ncov/hcp/clinical-care/-post-covid-conditions.html

4. Long COVID (Post-Acute Sequelae of SARS CoV-2 infection, PASC . Yale Medicine. Accessed August 28, 2022. https://www.yalemedicine.org/conditions/long-covid-post-acute-sequelae-of-sars-cov-2-infection-pasc.

5. Dani M, Dirksen A, Taraborrelli P, et al. Autonomic dysfunction in 'long COVID': rationale, physiology and management strategies. Clin Med

(Lond). 2021;21(1):e63–e67. doi:10.7861/clinmed-.2020-0896

6. PASC Dashboard. Accessed August 28, 2022. https://pascdashboard.aapmr.org
7. NIH | When COVID-19 Symptoms Linger. NIH COVID-19 Research. Updated August 13, 2021. Accessed August 28, 2022. https://-covid19.nih.gov/news-and-stories/when-COVID-19-symptoms-linger

8. Interim Guidance on Evaluating and Caring for Patients with Post-COVID Conditions. Centers for Disease Control and Prevention. Updated June 14, 2021. Accessed August 28, 2022. https://www.cdc.gov/coronavirus/2019-ncov/hcp/clinical-care/post-covid-index.html

9. Yomogida K, Zhu S, Rubino F, Figueroa W, Balanji N, Holman E. Post-Acute Sequelae of SARS-CoV-2 Infection Among Adults Aged ≥18 Years — Long Beach, California, April 1–December 10, 2020. MMWR Morb Mortal Wkly Rep 2021;70:1274–1277. DOI: http://dx.-doi.org/10.15585/mmwr.mm7037a2

10. Groff D, Sun A, Ssentongo AE, et al. Short-term and Long-term Rates of Postacute Sequelae of SARS-CoV-2 Infection: A Systematic Review. JAMA Netw Open. 2021;4(10):e2128568. doi:10.1001/jamanetworkopen.2021.28568

11. Coronavirus Disease (COVID-19): What Is It, Symptoms, Causes & Prevention. Cleveland Clinic. Updated March 1, 2022. Accessed August 28, 2022. https://my.clevelandclinic.org/health/diseases/21214-coronavirus-covid-19

12. Employment Development Department. State of California. Accessed August 28, 2022. https://www.edd.ca.gov/

13. Pleurisy: Causes, Symptoms, Diagnosis, Treatment & Prevention. Cleveland Clinic. August 16, 2022. Accessed August 28, 2022. https://my.clevelandclinic.org/health/diseases/21172-pleurisy

14. Pleurisy - Symptoms and causes. Mayo Clinic. Updated July 1, 2022. Accessed August 28, 2022. https://www.mayoclinic.org/diseases-conditions/pleurisy/symptoms-causes/syc-20351863

15. RECOVER: Researching COVID to Enhance Recovery. RECOVER. Accessed August 28, 2022. https://recovercovid.org

16. Electromyography (EMG): Testing, Muscle Weakness, Nerve Damage. Cleveland Clinic. Updated December 6, 2016. Accessed August 28, 2022. https://my.clevelandclinic.org/health/articles/4825-electromyograms

17. Patent Foramen Ovale (PFO). American Heart

Association. Updated March 31, 2017. Accessed August 28, 2022. https://www.heart.org/en/health-topics/congenital-heart-defects/about-congenital-heart-defects/patent-foramen-ovale-pfo

18. Patent Foramen Ovale (PFO): Symptoms, Causes & Treatment. Updated July 15, 2022. Accessed August 28, 2022.Cleveland Clinic. https://my.clevelandclinic.org/health/diseases/17326-patent-foramen-ovale-pfo

19. Patent foramen ovale - Symptoms and causes. Mayo Clinic. Updated September 2, 2021. Accessed August 28, 2022. https://www.mayoclinic.org/diseases-conditions/patent-foramen-ovale/symptoms-causes/syc-20353487

20. Factor V Leiden (FVL): Symptoms, Causes, Tests and Treatments. Cleveland Clinic. Updated April 16, 2019. Accessed August 28, 2022. https://my.clevelandclinic.org/health/diseases/17896-factor-v-leiden

21. Factor V Leiden - Symptoms and causes. Mayo Clinic. Updated August 23, 2022. Accessed August 28, 2022. https://www.mayoclinic.org/diseases-conditions/factor-v-leiden/symptoms-causes/syc-20372423

22. Transient ischemic attack (TIA) - Symptoms

and causes. Mayo Clinic. March 26, 2022. Accessed August 28, 2022. https://www.mayoclinic.org/diseases-conditions/transient-ischemic-attack/symptoms-causes/syc-20355679

23. What Does COVID Do to Your Blood? | Johns Hopkins Medicine. Updated March 3, 2022. Accessed August 28, 2022.https://www.hopkins-medicine.org/health/conditions-and-diseases/coronavirus/what-does-covid-do-to-your-blood

24. Demyelinating disease: What can you do about it? Mayo Clinic. Updated June 9.2022. Accessed August 28, 2022. www.mayoclinic.org/diseases-conditions/multiple-sclerosis/expert-answers/demyelinating-disease/faq-20058521.

About the Author

Shortly after writing this book, Dr. Salam Kabbani achieved her professional dream and accepted an infectious diseases pharmacist position at Olathe Medical Center in the greater Kansas City area. Shortly after that, she got COVID a THIRD time and was grateful to find the experience to be much lighter than the first two, leaving no lasting impact on her ability to resume her job. She is reconditioning her body and mind by taking swimming lessons, hiking as often as she can, and continuing to be an avid reader. She never takes anything for granted and knows that nothing is ever guaranteed, so she spends as much time as she can with her family, friends, and of course the beloved feline, Luna.

Acknowledgements

It takes a village to raise a child, and it certainly feels like it took a village to get me through this last year.

Mom : you never invalidated my pain, emotional or physical. You've been here for me through it all. You've tolerated my many mood swings, and sometimes I was so irritated with my symptoms, I took it out on you. You never left my side, even when I wasn't a little sweet pea. You've donated your time to travel with me and take me to all my appointments, which is truly the biggest gift of all.

Dad : you brought me medications when I couldn't get them myself, even though you were drowning in your own hectic physician schedule. You've paid for all my plane tickets to and from Cleveland and the many days of car rentals. Without your assistance, I would not have gotten my treatment.

Michelle : my angel of a next–door neighbor. You texted me every single day for 40 days to check in on me without knowing that this is the kind of connection I crave and need. No one else outside of my parents did that, and I will forever be indebted to your kindness. I'm sorry I gave you such grief about throwing out my trash. I should have just said yes.

Grandma and Uncle Amer : you let me stay with you for weeks on end while I was taking care of my health and never asked for anything in return. I know this will upset you guys because you think love should always be unconditional, but that's not the case for many people, so I need you both to know how much I love and appreciate you.

Patricia Carter, my healthcare provider : I am so blessed to be under your care. Thank you for continuously responding to my MyChart messages even now when I am having symptoms many months in. You are an incredible healer.

My family overseas : thank you for checking in on

me even when you had no water, heat, or electricity and were dealing with your own COVID infections. I don't know how you have the bandwidth to think of me, but you do, and I look forward to the day that I can visit you all.

My family in the USA : you have been so kind in checking on me, and you got me gifts! You made me feel so special and loved.

Osama: you chauffeured me all around Universal Studios and stood in so many lines to get me Butterbeer and Butterbeer ice cream. I will never be able to repay you.

My friends and colleagues that I regularly message with updates, **Amy Richardson, Barb Grajzl, Bhavin Mistry, Eric Myers, Grace Mitchell, Joann Taijala, Nicole Wilson, Samantha Ryan, and Raymond Vo**: you have made it all more palatable.

Dana, you are my best friend (no, it's not a tier): you have been there for me through it all. You check in on me regularly and you are constantly there for me. You go out of your way to make me feel loved and you notice details about me that no one else does. I am so lucky to have you in my life, and I hope you know how much I love you. I am grateful for our friendship every day.

Jennifer: I can't even put into words how much I love you. Adulting has proved to be challenging for all of us the last few years, and yet somehow you remember to message me on the exact days that I have provider appointments to make sure I know you are thinking of me. I don't know how you do it. I am so grateful for you and for the fact that pharmacy school brought us together.

Megan: you are one of a kind. Arguably the smartest person I know, and equally kind and loving to your friends, family, and patients. You are always there for me and go out of your way to see me and cook amazing meals when I visit. I love you.

Salam T: you will always be the other half to Salam–squared. The math is definitely wrong, but it will always be our inside joke. You made time to reach out to me during your medical school rotations and I will never forget that.

Stacy: you went from a preceptor to a close friend in a very short amount of time and you have allowed me to vent to you time and again with these symptoms. You've given so much advice, opened up your home to me, and let me partake in your family's holiday festivities. I love you.

Tammi: I don't even know where to begin. You are one of the kindest people I know, and I truly don't know how you do it all. You check in on me all the time despite everything going on in your own life, and I hope you know that I love you for it.

My cover reviewers and **everyone who's contributed to the production and development of this title** in some way : Thank you! I never imagined how much work goes into developing the perfect cover and choosing the right colors. I appreciate all your time and opinions very much!

My pharmacy technicians: you are wonderful people. You all continue to check in on me during my disability and I am just so blessed to have you all in my life. So many of us have gotten a COVID infection, but we will all continue to come out stronger.

My therapist: you can understand me better than I can understand myself sometimes, and you have and continue to help me get through every day.

My Bookstagram friends: you have been an online community of support. I never knew I could find so much kindness from people I have not met in real life, but many of you have been there for me and I am grateful for each and every one of you.

Jean Meltzer: I am so humbled to even have access to you, and I cannot tell you how much support and comfort you have provided me with. Your books alone made me feel seen, and even more so our many discussions filled with your insights and encouragement.

Lubna Allaf: I am so fortunate that we crossed paths at the Clinic. You were literally a guardian angel to me that day, and I know that forfeiting your lunch break to drive me in the wheelchair was not something you had planned on doing that day, but your kindness got me to my appointment.

My long–COVID community: you have made all the difference. Every transitional stage in this pandemic has been very scary for us, and for good reason. I am so grateful to have you all in my life.

The Cleveland Clinic: you make it possible for patients feeling helpless to come seek treatment from all around the world. Thank you for being a leader in healthcare and for having such an expansive insurance network. You make hope possible.

Dr. Sullivan: you are exceptional. You made me feel seen and heard. You removed a layer of isolation by sharing stories of other people with me. I hope to pass it forward by sharing my story with others.

Dr. Yost: your time in my life may have been very transient — six hours, to be exact — but you gave me the first glimpse of hope in a very long time.

Dr. Sharma: you gave me so much hope about the PFO closure, and when there didn't turn out to be a hole, you took the time to answer all my questions and help me understand a very perplexing medical circumstance. Thank you.

Dr. Wassif and Dr. Purpura: my time with you both was brief, but I appreciate every piece of advice that you offered, and I'm glad that you were a part of my journey.

Tim: you know how much your physical therapy guidance improved my health because you saw it first-hand. You helped me regain my strength. You helped me take control of my POTS. I continue to do my exercises almost every day, and if I ever get COVID again, I now know how to rehabilitate my muscles thanks to you.

Kaitlin: your clamshell exercises continue to kick my butt ... thank you! If you hadn't done that questionnaire and recommended speech therapy to me, I don't know where I'd be right now. I am forever indebted to you. You are so empathetic and nurturing, and I really appreciate that about you.

Abigail and Kayla: my two amazing speech therapists. You both have made such a difference in my life. You helped me refocus my memory, tolerate normal noises, regain control of my schedule, and basically be a functional human again. Thank you both for the amazing work that you do.

My editor, **Brooke Crites**: I'm so glad I found you in this chaotic literary world. You have provided me with very insightful feedback, and my book wouldn't be where it's at if it weren't for you.

My publisher, colleague, friend, and mentor, **Janan Sarwar**: I don't even know where to begin. You have been an incredible sounding board through this whole process. You have allowed me to be vulnerable with you, you've been vulnerable with me, and I really can't describe how much of a positive influence you've been in my life and on this book. You continue to give so many people voices, and I'm honored that you chose mine to be heard and shared.

Cory Jenks, I can only imagine your work as a pharmacist and comedian are as great as you say they are, because you reviewed my book, and oh look, it got published! In all seriousness, thank you for assisting with this process and helping us navigate the unknown references situation. You inspire me and countless other pharmacists to reach our respective potentials every day!

NOTES

....

....

....

....

....

....

....

....

....

....

....

....

....

....